WOULD YOU TEACH A FISH TO CLIMB A TREE?

A DIFFERENT TAKE ON KIDS WITH ADD, ADHD, OCD, AND AUTISM

WOULD YOU TEACH A FISH TO CLIMB A TREE?

~

A Different Take on Kids with ADD, ADHD, OCD, and Autism

By Anne Maxwell, LCSW,
Gary M. Douglas, and Dr. Dain Heer

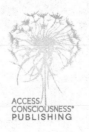

ACCESS
CONSCIOUSNESS®
PUBLISHING

Would You Teach a Fish to Climb a Tree?
A Different Take on Kids with ADD, ADHD, OCD, and Autism

Copyright © 2014 by Anne Maxwell,
Gary M. Douglas, and Dr. Dain Heer

ISBN: 978-1-939261-50-2

Interior Design: Karin Kinsey

Published by Access Consciousness Publishing, LLC

www.accessconsciousnesspublishing.com

Printed in the United States of America
International printing in the U.K. and Australia

First Edition

Everybody is a genius. But if you judge a fish by its ability to climb a tree, it will live its whole life believing that it is stupid.
~Albert Einstein

GRATITUDE

Great thanks to Jill McCormick for inspiring the writing of this book and for her many contributions that made it possible.

And to all the kids who have done our classes, special thanks for showing us the gift that you are, how we can help you, and how we might be able to have what you have.

CONTENTS

A WORD ABOUT LABELS

Don't define these children by their labels.
You will cut off your receiving of what they have to gift to you.
Instead ask a question,
"What is the gift they have that I am not receiving?"

~ Gary Douglas

Anne:
It has become increasingly clear to me over the years I have spent working with kids and families that there are particular "cultures" of thinking or attitude with regard to the way people—and especially kids—should function. Those who don't function according to the rules and regulations in play around them are labeled by the advocates and promoters of those "cultures." This tends to happen a great deal in educational and medical communities.

So often the conclusion is reached that children who don't "fit in" need to be taught how to behave so they can learn to function as if they were "normal" and "average" and just like everyone else. The problem is that they are *not* normal and average. My point of view is that by asking them to be normal and average, we are doing two things: We are telling them that there is something wrong with them, and we are asking them to become someone they are not.

Labels evoke images, answers, and definitions, and nothing can be considered that doesn't fit within the confines of the labels. In other words, the labels define, and once one is labeled, he or she is always labeled! Some of the most commonly used labels are autism, OCD, ADD, and ADHD. In the medical community, all of these diagnoses are described in varying intensity, from mild to severe.

Autism Spectrum Disorders. There is a group of mental health diagnoses that fall under the generic category of Autism Spectrum Disorders, or ASD. These include Autistic Disorder, Asperger's Syndrome, and Pervasive Developmental Disorder. These diagnoses attempt to describe a variety of symptoms, skills, and difficulties people have with functioning in this reality. People who have been diagnosed with ASD are sometimes referred to as "being on the spectrum." They function differently from so-called normal people with regard to communication, social interaction, and relationships. Their behaviors tend to be repetitive and can appear "odd" and the severity of their symptoms range from those of highly functional people to individuals who are not able to speak or function in this reality.

Obsessive Compulsive Disorder, or OCD, is a diagnosis that describes recurrent and persistent thought patterns and behaviors that are repetitive and ritualistic and cause enough distress that they can interfere with daily life.

Then, there are the diagnoses of **Attention Deficit Disorder,** or ADD, and **Attention Deficit Hyperactivity Disorder,** or ADHD. People with these diagnoses tend to have difficulty paying attention to just one thing; they appear not to be listening, and they are easily distracted. Those with ADHD tend to be extremely active. They are often unable to remain seated, and their behaviors include fidgeting, squirming in their seats, talking excessively, impulsively blurting out answers, and interrupting.

ADD, ADHD, OCD, and autism are among the labels that can "sentence" a child to being thought of in a certain way. These labels are known to describe "disabilities," and kids with those diagnoses are defined and viewed as "disabled" or "handicapped." It does not seem as if there is room for any other way of thinking about them once that judgment has been made.

I am aware of how hopeless it can be for those who do not fit into the culture and who are branded and classified as disabled, impaired, or defective. This also applies to the parents of these kids who would like so much for their children to have happy, successful lives.

There are, however, more and more stories in the popular press about kids who were diagnosed with autism at an early age and whose parents were told they would never read, talk, or relate to people. These kids are now in their early teens and are doing undergraduate and graduate level classes in major universities. What's the common thread in those stories? It is the parents who didn't buy the labels that were placed on their kids and instead recognized that so much more was possible than what the experts told them.

These parents encouraged their children to follow their interests and do what they loved to do, no matter how odd it may have seemed. A particularly inspiring story was told by a mother whose autistic son just wanted to play with shapes and shadows. He was failing in his "Special Ed" program, where he was being forced to do things he didn't want to do. She found that the more she encouraged him to do what he enjoyed, the more his shell cracked open. And when she followed his interests and made resources available to him to support those interests, he began to talk and to thrive.

When he was three years old, she was told that he would never talk. At eleven years of age, he enrolled in a university and began studying mathematics.

~ 2 ~

A NEW PERSPECTIVE

What if there's nothing wrong with these kids?
What if they are just different?
- Gary Douglas

Anne:

My first job out of graduate school in 1991, as a child and family therapist, was at a residential treatment center for kids who were labeled with psychiatric disorders. These were kids who were unable to function at home, in school, or in the community and had "failed" multiple times in less restrictive settings. In the United States, residential treatment centers are considered to be almost the end of the road for kids. The only places further down that road are jails or state mental hospitals.

There were two ways for kids to be at the center—in the residential program, meaning they lived in one of the residential units 24/7 and attended the highly specialized school program as well—or in the day treatment program, which meant they lived off-campus and attended the highly specialized school program during the school week. I was hired as a psychotherapist in both the residential and day treatment programs, and I worked with kids between the ages of three and eighteen. My specialty was the younger ones.

The kids who were diagnosed with ADD, ADHD, OCD, and autism were the ones who presented challenges of a different sort to the staff. Many were in constant motion, even when sitting in chairs. They laughed at all the (seemingly) wrong times and blurted out answers but couldn't explain how they got them, even when the answers were correct. The behavioral program had little to no effect on these kids. They were viewed as disrespectful, oppositional, difficult, and hard to work with. Others, who were more severely disabled, seemed pretty checked out and shut down. When they did respond, they seemed to be reacting to something not apparent to the rest of us. Sometimes they became enraged with what appeared to be little to no provocation. Their emotional outbursts had an intensity about them that straightened my spine!

There was a wide range of people on staff at the center, and they came from many different disciplines. My favorites were the magical ones who saw the kids for who they were, not as the labels they had been given. They were the people who gave the kids the benefit of the doubt. They knew the kids were doing the best they could with the tools they had. And these were the people the kids liked best. One of those magical people was a woman named Naomi, who was a specialist in the school program. When I met Naomi, I was fresh out of grad school and I felt a particular kinship for kids who had difficulties concentrating and focusing. I asked her about kids with ADD and ADHD. She said, "It's like they have hundreds of television screens in their heads and each screen is tuned in to a different channel. The volume is turned up and they don't have a remote to turn it down or switch all the screens to the same channel. They can't help it!"

That made sense to me. At times, it seemed like the kids tried so hard to focus and concentrate yet they seemed utterly incapable of doing so. I felt a connection with them because I too have always had several things going on in my head at the same time. As a child, I was always being told to pay attention. I'd often wonder what was wrong with me that I couldn't do that.

In the program, there was an emphasis on medications, and great value was placed on being able to sit still and listen. It was always clear when the meds went too far in the opposite direction and the kids focused on what they were doing to the exclusion of everything around them, and for example, colored so intently that the colored markers went through the paper. With heavy doses of medications, it seemed as if the kids became flat. Their sparkle was gone.

Naomi had some suggestions that worked with the kids. For example, she told me, "If you can't say what needs to be said in five words or less, they won't hear you." It was true. Their eyes would glaze over at anything more. However, as useful as Naomi's suggestions were, they weren't enough to make a real or lasting difference with the kids. What she didn't tell me—and what neither of us knew at the time—is that their minds moved at the speed of light. Words were not their preferred form of communication because words were too painfully slow, laborious, and difficult. Although I did not know this way back then, I now realize that they communicated primarily energetically.

Fast forward to twenty years later when I met Gary Douglas, the founder of Access Consciousness®. He put into words what I had known secretly about these kids for so long but had never given myself permission to acknowledge, as it flew in the face of what was considered real and true at the time. When he said that kids who have been diagnosed with ADD, ADHD, OCD, and/or autism become angry when they are told to use words because words slow them down so much, a great sense of relief washed through me. Memories of so many different kids throwing tantrums at the center, and later in my private practice, came back to me. I recalled the looks of utter disdain that crossed their faces when they were told to use their words or when someone said, "I didn't hear you." It made so much sense to me—because these kids do communicate differently.

When Gary asked questions like "What if there's nothing wrong with these kids?" and "What if they are just different?" I thought to myself, "Finally, someone who gets it!" What if kids with all those labels could be seen as who they are—not as who they aren't? What could that change?

Gary's comments invited me to begin asking questions like "What else is possible here that we're not looking at?" rather than "How can we make this child fit in?"

What if different is different—not right, not wrong—just *different*? These kids aren't the same as other people. They don't have emotions the way other people do. They think differently. They don't understand why people move so slowly and pretend not to know what they actually *do* know. They have a different way of looking at the world. And what if they actually have special talents and abilities?

A ten-year-old boy who had been diagnosed with OCD was in my office the other day. He feels so different from other kids and so *wrong*. We were talking in a relaxed way and enjoying ourselves. Then I noticed a subtle change in his body. He looked at me, looked at the telephone on the desk behind me, looked at me again, and then the phone rang. I raised my eyebrows and smiled at him, and he smiled back.

"You knew it was going to ring, didn't you?" I asked.

He giggled. "Yes!"

"Awesome!" I replied.

What if *we* could see what *they* see, rather than try to get *them* to see what *we* see? What change could that create?

What's created by not acknowledging the abilities these kids have? I believe it causes them to see themselves as invisible, not deserving, unworthy, not good enough, defective, weird, and wrong. What if that is the harm that we do to kids who are diagnosed with the labels ADD, ADHD, OCD, and autism? They don't see the world the same way we do, and when we won't see through their eyes, that creates difficulties for them. We need to see what they see rather than try to get them to see things our way.

~ 3 ~
WHAT IF YOUR CHILDREN ARE PERFECT?

What if your children are perfect—even if they have ADHD, OCD, ADD, autism, or something else going on?
- Dr. Dain Heer

Gary:

Dain and I have had the opportunity to work with some children who have been labeled with these so-called disabilities. Initially, we tried to deal with these conditions from the point of view that something was wrong with the kids, and we tried to figure out how we could handle their "disability." However, in the process of working with a number of great kids, we've seen that they have many abilities, talents, and gifts that go unrecognized by teachers, parents, and people in the medical and psychological community.

People tend to function from the point of view that there is something wrong with these children because they don't learn the way the rest of us do. The reality is that they pick things up in a totally different manner, and we need to step up and find out how they learn, not try to teach them using methods that might have worked for us but definitely don't work for them.

We would like to re-reference the point of view that they are "special needs" children; they are actually special *talents* children. We call them X-Men, after the Marvel Comic superhero team composed of mutants with an X-gene who use their extra powers and abilities for the benefit of humanity. For us, it's a term of affection. The X-Men are here with us on the planet to make waves. They are a mutation that is an expansion of the species, but they are being looked at as though they are a limitation. We don't believe that is true.

We would like to unlock the abilities these kids have because it is our perception that if they were given the opportunity, they might be able to change many of the things on our planet that will turn into disasters in the future.

We ask that you don't see your kids as wrong, no matter what they've been labeled. Look at your kids not from the wrongness of them but from the rightness of them. When you do this, you can create a completely different world for yourself, for them, and for everyone on the planet. We hope you will see that you have an extraordinary opportunity to create a more conscious world. You can create a place in which people begin to see the ability and the greatness these kids are.

CREATING A CULTURE OF QUESTION

The purpose of question is to create awareness.
- Gary Douglas

Anne:

So many of the parents who come to see me find themselves at a complete loss as to how to assist their children. Some of them buy into the conclusion that there is something "wrong" with their child. Many of them extrapolate that "wrongness" to themselves. They believe that somehow they *did* something wrong or that they *are* intrinsically wrong. How else could they have had a child like this? Many of them voice shame and guilt over what they perceive as their seemingly diminished capacities as parents. And most of them try to figure it all out by trying to find the answer that explains why their child is the way he or she is. They tell me that if they could only *understand,* they would know what to do.

What if these kids are not their labels? Instead of buying into any labeling that is done to these kids, what if we could ask questions instead? Let's talk for a minute about questions. I love the description of question that Gary gives: A question is not a statement with a question mark at the end of it. A question is a question. Unlike what we are taught in school, the purpose of a question is not to find "the right answer." The purpose of a question is to create awareness.

Dain:

The question is the key to opening other doorways of possibility.

Anne:

"What do you want for dinner?" Is that a question or a statement with a question mark at the end of it? It's a statement with a question mark at the end of it because it presupposes a) that the person is hungry, b) that he plans on eating, and c) that what he eats will be in the form of dinner.

"Are you hungry?" That's a question. It opens the door to possibilities.

Asking real questions is one of the most amazing tools of Access Consciousness. I find that by asking a question, I am able —instantly—to step out of the density of whatever conclusion or point of view is trapping me and into the space of possibilities and choice.

The mother of six-year-old twins, a boy and a girl, came to see me at the start of the school year. She is brilliant, as is her husband. She and her daughter function with greater ease socially than her husband or her son do. The mother and daughter are more outgoing and talkative; the father and son are more quiet, and some might say, withdrawn.

She came to see me because her son was struggling with his first grade program. Reports from the teacher stated that he was acting out, throwing tantrums, not focusing on his work, and "isolating" during recess. When the boy arrived home after school, he was irritable, fussy, argumentative, and whiny, and his mother would know that it was just a matter of time before he would throw a tantrum. She was well aware of how different her son was, and although she privately acknowledged his considerable talents and abilities, she found herself apologizing to the school staff for his behavior. All she could see was what wasn't working, and the conclusions she reached were propelling her into a state of despair and hopelessness. She said to me, "It's only the first month of first grade. He's got twelve more years of school to go!"

I asked her several questions:

- What do you know about your son that you are not acknowledging?
- What are his strengths?
- What does your son require in order to thrive in school?
- If he could design his school experience this year, what would it be?
- What does he know that you're not asking about or acknowledging?

The questions allowed her to go beyond needing to come up with answers and move into the space of being aware of what she did know about her son, the school, and herself. When she let go of needing to have an answer to justify or prove something about him, she lightened up considerably. She realized she knew far more about her situation than she had given herself credit for. For example, she acknowledged that her son functioned academically far beyond the rest of his classmates and probably was excruciatingly bored. She was able to approach the staff at the school, and together they designed a program for her son. The boy was transitioned into the second grade and was given challenging work at even higher grade levels for many of the subjects. His tantrums and outbursts reduced significantly.

She also stopped worrying about how he "isolated" during recesses and acknowledged that he probably benefited from having some time by himself. She recognized that he was less social than his sister—and that was okay. As a result, she saw his brilliance in using some time alone as a way of managing the over-stimulation of school and school recesses.

By stepping out of the world of judgment and right or wrong answers, she created a culture of question around her son's experience at school, which allowed everyone involved to see the possibilities and different choices that come with awareness.

Tool: What Is This?

Here are four beautiful all-purpose questions I learned from Gary that every parent can use:

- What is this?
- What can I do with it?
- Can I change it?
- How can I change it?

The mother of two boys, ages five and three, told me she was at a loss as to how to handle her five year old. Although he had not been diagnosed with ADHD, she believed that he had many of the symptoms. He was impulsive and easily excitable, and he was not well-liked by kids his age because he flew off the handle so easily.

She said that recently, she picked him up from his preschool and took him to soccer practice. After that, she ran some errands with him and his brother. They went to the bank first and then to the grocery store. As they were leaving the grocery store, it started to rain hard, and even though they ran, they were soaking wet by the time they got in the car. She had one towel, and as she dried the three year old, they giggled together. Then, as she attempted to dry off the five year old, he started to scream at her. "Nooooo! Dooooon't! I don't want that towel!"

I asked her, "Did he ask to be dried off?"

"No," she replied, "but he was sopping wet!"

In a previous session, I had presented these four questions to her. I said, "What if you asked yourself, 'What is this? What can I do with it? Can I change it? How can I change it?' Start with 'What is this?' When you ask it, what do you get?"

"I don't know! I was just trying to help him out. He was so over the top! He gets like that and I don't know what to do."

I asked, "What if it had nothing to do with being wet? What if you were using the wrong towel?" I repeated, "What was that?"

She said, "He just gets so mad at me!"

I asked, "What is he mad about, beyond being dried with the towel?"

"Well, I suppose he was tired and hungry."

I asked, "Does he get any down time?"

She said, "Well, I try to get everything done. I'm kind of a perfectionist. I want everything to be right."

"So, what can you do with that information—that he's tired and hungry and you have an agenda to get stuff done?"

She paused before responding, "I get that I push him pretty hard to keep up with me."

I asked, "Can you change it? How can you change it?"

She said, "Well, I could not pack so much stuff in. I could take him home and let him decompress. I guess that preschool, then soccer, then errands is a lot."

I asked, "Do you play with him?"

Marcus

One of my friends, a school speech pathologist who works in the public school system, tells this story about one of her students:

Marcus was ten years old. He had been diagnosed with cerebral palsy and had been in a wheelchair from the time he was tiny. He had never walked or talked. He was a joyful little boy, who, rather than moving and talking, engaged her with facial expressions. She told me that his joyfulness and total lack of sadness about his condition led her to ask the question, "What if this condition isn't a travesty?" She then asked other questions like "What if my target today is to create as much joy and possibility in his universe as can be generated? What if that became my priority over trying to get him to function like all the other kids?"

She said that as soon as she began to ask questions and let go of her point of view that it was wrong for a child to have the kind of challenge Marcus had, possibilities for him began to show up that she hadn't seen before. Their interactions became playful and fun, and he began to enjoy his time with her even more.

One day she told him, "We are going to find a way for you to talk." She started using augmentative communication devices that assist people who have difficulties with spoken and written language. She said that her training told her that because Marcus had cerebral palsy, he wasn't supposed to be able to speak or comprehend what she was saying. However, she told me that over time, he actually began to vocalize and make sounds.

Then, one day, when she was at the chalk board doing a lesson in colors, she asked, "What color is this?"

She said, "Somewhere behind me I heard the word green. I turned to see Marcus smiling at the back of the classroom. He did it! Not only did he say the word green. Green was the right answer!"

"Not very much. I'm usually pretty busy."

"Anything there you could change?"

She laughed. "I guess so!"

I spoke with her the following week. She told me she had rearranged her schedule so that her son had more "time off," and she was making a point of playing with him each day, even if it was just for a little while. She said that life in their house was much easier now; he was happier, and she was less driven to "get stuff done."

All because she asked some questions.

~ 5 ~
WE'RE ALL INFINITE BEINGS
THAT MEANS YOUR KIDS ARE TOO

It's important to acknowledge what kids know and what they are aware of, even when they're very young. They are infinite beings even if their bodies are small.

~ Gary Douglas

Gary:

Let's start out by talking about the fact that we're all infinite beings. Each one of us is an infinite being, and as an infinite being, we have the infinite capacity to perceive everything, know everything, be everything, and receive everything. We can function from total awareness and total consciousness in all aspects of our life—if we choose to do so.

One of the greatest gifts you can give yourself is to recognize that in your child, you have a small body and an infinite being. That being, your child, knows things, perceives things, and receives things. You need to acknowledge that and not try to come from the perspective that you're superior because you're an adult. Your kids are infinite beings too, and even though their bodies are smaller than yours, it doesn't mean *they* are smaller than you are.

Anne:

Exactly! Some questions I ask parents are:

- What if children know more than you think they know?
- What if you asked them what they know—and what contribution they could be to you?

Oftentimes parents will bring their infants and/or toddlers to sessions with me when they come to talk about older siblings. Or couples will come in because their marriage isn't working the way they would like and they will bring an infant or toddler along. It's amazing to see what the kids "know" and the contribution they are in the session.

The other day, a couple came to see me for the first time. They wanted to discuss their marriage, and they brought their son, who is eleven months old. He sat on his mom's lap, staring at me for a while before venturing onto the floor to examine the toys. He continued to look at me as the session progressed and moved closer and closer to my chair. Finally, he was sitting so close he was leaning up against my legs. At one point, during a particularly heated moment between his parents, he turned around and tried to climb into my lap. I picked him up, and he sat there, watching his parents and turning slightly to check my face. It was as if he was telling his parents, "You don't have to stay stuck here. You can let it go!" As his parents began to move beyond the place in which they had battled, he indicated to me that he was ready to get back down and play on the floor again, which he did, ever aware of what was transpiring. Periodically he went over to them, and standing up next to their legs, looked at them. He wasn't asking for attention; he was simply being present with them as they worked through their "stuff."

He was so present and so aware of the turmoil his parents had been creating as well as the shift that occurred when they chose to be in a different space. He was an amazing contribution to his parents, whether they acknowledged it or not. Little body? Yes, absolutely. He's learning how to walk, he doesn't yet speak with words, his coordination is awkward, and yet none of that prevents him from knowing *exactly* what is going on.

Gary:

So often adults assume that because kids are young or have small bodies, they are unaware or unintelligent and need to be diminished, controlled, and told what to do. People see them as too young or too disabled to understand what's going on, or they make rules about what they can and cannot do—without any regard for the infinite being in front of them. This may be part of what we see in autistic kids and the anger that comes from them when their infinite capacity to perceive, know, be, and receive everything is not acknowledged.

Anne:

It infuriates them to be talked down to or patronized. When parents, other adults, or older siblings put themselves in a position of superiority over kids that we refer to as the X-Men, the kids tend to become angry. What if *they* don't view themselves as inferior? Autistic kids perceive so much, and they can become extremely frustrated when they have difficulty communicating that information to the people around them. They do take in information differently, and when people judge them or look down on them, they don't like it!

A great question that I first heard from Dain and now ask parents and kids is:

- What do you know that you're pretending not to know or denying that you know, that if you could acknowledge it, would change everything?

This question bypasses the logical thinking brain and goes straight to the energy of whatever is causing you to be stuck. It creates awareness of what is actually going on. And it's a question that you can pose to babies and toddlers as well as older children and adults. It doesn't require a verbal response, although sometimes there is one. It's amazing to see the shifts that can occur after asking it.

A brilliant nine-year-old boy who had been diagnosed with ADHD and could also be diagnosed with mild autism was struggling in school. He and his mother were at war with teachers, administrators, and peers—and it was a war for control. When I asked him, "What do you know that you're pretending not to know or denying that you know, that if you could acknowledge it, would change everything?" his eyes rolled to the back of his head and he said, "That's the stupidest question I ever heard!" He then proceeded to tell me for the next thirty minutes how the school functioned and how specific teachers and administrators operated. He also acknowledged that he could make different choices rather than being at war with them…if he chose. The question gave him the awareness that was required for him to begin to change the way he approached the school and his teachers. And when we told his mom what he had told me, her son's awareness freed her up so she was able to approach the school in a way that was a contribution rather than a confrontation, which is where she had been stuck.

Infinite beings function from the space of awareness. When you stop looking for answers about and for these kids and instead seek greater awareness of what they know and what they actually require, things change. This doesn't mean that you, as an adult, don't know anything. Of course you do. What I'm suggesting is that you can change the energy of a situation and invite a totally different outcome when you ask, "What contribution can I be to my child?" Doesn't that have a different energy from telling him things or trying to control him? And what if you could also ask, "What contribution could I receive from my child?" You may be like the parents of the toddler in my office who were able to receive their child's contribution, even though they might not have been aware that's what they were doing.

Gary:

Acknowledging that kids—all kids—are infinite beings with an infinite ability to perceive, know, be, and receive everything is the single most important thing that you, as a parent or a teacher, can do to assist them to access their talents and capacities. This is especially true for kids with autism, OCD, ADD, ADHD and all those other labels—because they have special gifts.

Anne:

One of the mistakes people make is assuming that because kids are little, they don't know anything or they are not aware.

A grandmother brought her four-year-old granddaughter to see me. The girl was easily agitated at preschool and had nightmares at night. She slept in her grandmother's king-sized bed, wrapped around her grandmother's body.

The girl's mother had been brutally murdered by a boyfriend, and the grandmother had not wanted her granddaughter to know about the crime because it had been so gruesome and the girl was so young. She told the girl that her mom had gotten sick and the doctors had tried to save her but couldn't fix her.

A few months after the girl had been in play therapy with me, her grandmother told me that she was asking her how her mother had died. "She tells me the kids at school want to know how her mama died. I don't know what to say to her. I can't tell her what happened."

I asked her, "What if you ask her what she knows?" Grandmother initially refused, insisting once again that the murder had been so horrible and her granddaughter was too young.

The girl persisted, and one day her grandmother did ask her, "What do you know about how Mama died?"

In four-year-old language, the girl accurately described in great detail *exactly* how her mother had been murdered.

Grandmother was stunned. "How did you know?" she asked.

"Gamma, he told me and he told Mama and he told the dog he would do that to us." She then repeated what the murderer's threats had been.

Grandmother told her, "What he did was *very* bad, and he's going to spend the rest of his life locked up in jail. The judge says he can never get out. He can never come and hurt you."

That night, the girl slept on her side of the bed for the first time since her mother's death, and within a few days, she was sleeping in her own bedroom again.

All this from acknowledging that her granddaughter was an infinite being rather than a child who was too young to know anything—and then asking the simple question, "What do you know?"

6

WHAT A WOLF SHOWED US ABOUT HOW KIDS WITH AUTISM COMMUNICATE

When you understand how kids with autism communicate, your communication with them can go to a place that allows you— and them—to have much greater ease.

~ Dr. Dain Deer

Gary:

I have done a lot of work with animals, especially horses, but also with dogs and other four-legged creatures, because animals will talk to me.

One day a lady called me and said, "I have a problem with my wolf. I'm getting ready to take a trip, and he has become very anxious. I keep trying to calm him down. I tell him that everything is going to be okay, that I'm going away and I'll be back, but he gets more and more frantic every day."

I said, "I'll see if I can work with him."

I went to her ranch and I asked, "What's going on, Mr. Wolf?" and he downloaded an incredible amount of information to me.

I said, "Slow down. I can't understand that. It's too fast for me."

He slowed it down and I began to get his pictures. He let me know that the lady had been telling him that she was going to go away and that she would come back, and not to worry.

I asked him, "What does that mean to you?" and he showed me her dying. He thought she was saying that she was going to die and she would come back in another body, because that had happened before. She had died, all the wolves mourned her, and then at a later time, she came back in another body.

This was the first wolf I had ever dealt with, and I was surprised by his capacity to download information. I didn't know this was a capability wolves had. I had thought he would have a more dog-like reality.

I reassured him that the lady was not going to die; she was simply going away for a couple of weeks and she would be back. Our conversation calmed him down. He stopped pacing and following the woman around the house. He started eating again and resumed his normal sleep habits. The woman was able to take her trip without worrying about him.

A few weeks after I worked with the wolf, Dain asked me to help him work with a lady and her autistic son.

Dain:
A woman called and asked, "Could you work on me and my four-year-old son, Nicolas?"

I said, "Sure, no problem. What's going on?"

She said, "He is autistic. He only has a vocabulary of forty words."

I said, "That will be a new one for me. Let's see what shows up."

Then I asked Gary, "Can you come and work with us?" and he said, "Yes."

In the course of working with Nicolas, Gary realized that Nicolas downloaded information to him just like the wolf did. It was an instantaneous download, like playing an entire movie in a split second. Nicolas downloaded the whole movie all at once. Not frame one, frame two, frame three, and so forth. For someone who is autistic, that would be so painful.

Gary:

We worked with Nicolas for about an hour. He learned one new word, and we learned an amazing amount of information about autistic children. One of the things we discovered is that autistic children don't have a separation between past, present, and future. For them, everything is here and now.

At one point, Nicolas' mother said to us, "I think my son is one of my grandparents."

I asked, "Really, which one?"

She said, "I think he is my grandfather."

I asked, "What was your grandfather's name?"

She said, "Bill."

I turned to Nicolas. He was facing the window, looking out onto the horizon. I said "Bill," and he instantly turned around and locked eyes with me. For those of you who may not know about autistic children, they don't like to make eye contact. It's difficult for them to do that, and it rarely occurs.

Dain:

Throughout the time we spent with Nicolas and his mother, we had often said Nicolas' name, but he never made any response at all. It was very interesting to see the way he responded to the name *Bill*. It was also very interesting the way Nicolas learned to say the word *jump*.

Gary:

Nicolas was climbing up onto a footstool and jumping off it, and because I realized that he was communicating telepathically, I wanted to see if giving him a picture of jumping at the same time I said the word *jump* might help him to learn the word.

After I did that a couple of times, he said, "Jump."

When we finished working together, Nicolas went to the door and started banging on the handle. His mother kept saying, "Nicolas, come over here, put your shoes on, go. Put your shoes on, put your shoes on."

Remembering what I had learned from the wolf, I said to her, "He is not getting the steps the way you're breaking them down. You have to download the whole picture of his leaving the door, walking over to you, sitting down, putting on his shoes, letting you tie them, taking your hand, and the two of you walking out the door."

She asked, "How do I do that?"

I said, "There's no *how*. Just do it."

She did, and Nicolas instantaneously left the door, went over to her, and sat down. She put on his shoes and tied them. He took her hand and led her to the door.

Dain:

It was like running a whole movie all at once and saying, "Here you go. Here's the whole movie."

Gary:

This is the way these children communicate. They are psychic or telepathic or whatever you want to call it. They get the whole picture at once—but rather than being aware of how their world functions, we keep trying to make them slow down and function in our step-by-step world.

Dain:

I called Nicolas' mother about two months after we worked with Nicolas to see how they were doing. She said, "Well, we were doing great, but over the past ten days, Nicolas has been getting worse. I don't know what's wrong! He has started to exhibit almost every sign of autism."

I asked, "What's going on? What has changed?"

She said, "I don't know."

I asked, "Have you been doing anything differently?"

She said, "Well, over the last ten days or so, I've been researching the symptoms of autism on the Internet."

I said, "Do you remember that we told you how psychic and aware Nicolas is? And how he doesn't have past, present, and future? He's all awareness. He is willing to pick up everything out of your head. You are reading up on the symptoms of autism, and he's picking them up out of your head and manifesting them. Will you do me a favor and stop today?"

She said, "But I have to do this research."

I said, "No, you don't. You have to be with your kid, and you have to stop screwing him up with what's going on in your head."

She said, "Okay, I'll try it."

When I checked back with her, things had returned to normal. She gave up researching autism on the Internet, just to see what would happen, and Nicolas stopped exhibiting all the symptoms she had been reading about.

Gary:

A few months later, we did an X-Men class in Houston, and she brought Nicolas. I asked her, "How does Nicolas do on a playground?"

She said, "Oh, there's no problem on the playground. He plays with other children."

I asked, "Really? Does he talk to them?"

She said, "No, but they seem to do whatever he wants. He is always the leader."

Dain:

He just communicates with pictures to the other kids and they don't have any barriers to communicating in that way.

Gary:

The mother of another autistic boy we worked with said a similar thing. I asked her if she had any other kids and she said, yes, she had another boy and a girl. I asked how the autistic boy did with his brother.

She said, "Oh, he is great with his brother. They play just fine."

I asked, "Are you aware that they communicate telepathically?"

She said, "What do you mean?"

I asked, "Do you hear them talking?"

She said, "No, never." She hadn't noticed that these two boys played without ever speaking. They were communicating telepathically. That's what these kids are capable of.

I'd be willing to bet that if you have an autistic child, you have been communicating telepathically with your child and didn't even notice. They put things in your head. They will say, "Go" and you'll say, "I'm going now." They will say, "I'm hungry," and you will ask, "What would you like to eat?" A lot of kids do this sort of thing before they learn to speak.

A lady in Australia brought her autistic nephew and his mother to see me at my friend Simone's house. We were standing in the kitchen and I was trying to tap into the boy's head to see what was going on for him. All of a sudden, his mother asked Simone, "Do you have any juice?"

Simone said, "Yeah, there is some in the refrigerator. Help yourself."

The woman walked over to the refrigerator and asked her son, "Billy, would you like some juice?"

I said, "Hold on a minute. Are you aware that he is standing in front of the refrigerator and he knows what is in there? He put it into your head to get juice for him, and now you are asking him if wants some. You have to get clear. This kid communicates telepathically with you."

The mother nodded and smiled. As soon as I said it to her, she knew it was true.

Dain:

Your kids will think a question at you and you'll answer it—and you'll never even notice that your child didn't speak. If you decide the only way to communicate with your child is for your child to learn to speak, you won't be able to see that there is a whole world of communication available to you. You have to start paying attention to when kids think things at you and the information that comes through—because although you may not yet know it, you can communicate with them. You have the same abilities they do.

7

COMMUNICATING WITH PICTURES

Have you ever had the experience of dreading something—going to a meeting, getting everybody out of the house on time, or putting the kids to bed—and it turned out to be just as difficult as you knew it would? What if you and everyone else involved were sending each other the pictures that created that situation?
~ Anne Maxwell

Anne:

Many parents I've worked with have said that mornings are difficult. The mom of a seven-year-old girl who had been diagnosed with mild autism told me that from the minute the alarm went off in the morning, an energy of dread swept over her and the entire household, and true to form, mornings typically were difficult, with tantrums, upsets, anger, drama, and nothing getting done. She told me that she would break down tasks, as she had been coached to do, giving her daughter first one thing to do, then when that was done, another thing. However, she acknowledged that it didn't work—to the point that nothing was getting done, not even the first task. And everyone in the family became upset.

We talked about sending pictures instead of verbally breaking down tasks for her daughter to do. I asked her to recall a morning that had gone smoothly and to tap into the energy of what that morning had been like. I then asked her to send her daughter, the other kids, and her husband a "picture" of the energy of things getting done with peace and ease. She did, and she said that mornings changed almost immediately.

Weeks later she called to thank me, and to let me know that she was sending pictures to her daughter whether the girl was in her presence or not, and that sending pictures from a distance worked "pretty well." She said her daughter was getting lots more done in the mornings, and that the mornings, and indeed the rest of the days, were so much easier. She told me that she wasn't telling, re- minding, or nagging her daughter to do things any more, and it was creating much more ease between the two of them.

Gary:

Sometimes you communicate with pictures without even realiz- ing it, just because you have the intention for your child to under- stand you. I talked with a parent in Australia, who said, "When my daughter, who is autistic, was younger, she was very anxious about anything that was new. If we were going to do something different, we had to explain it to her. And as all adults know, it's often very dif- ficult to explain something new to a small child. I'd say, 'We have to go to Perth.' She would ask, 'What's Perth?' and on and on it went. I think that without knowing it, I began to put things in pictures, because halfway through our conversation, she would say, 'Oh yeah, I remember. It's okay.'"

Anne:

One mom told me that she sent pictures to her son of giving her a hug when she got home at the end of the day—and he did. Another mom told me that she sent pictures to her teenage daughter of hav- ing a clean, picked-up bedroom, and lo and behold, the daughter picked up her bedroom that weekend.

Gary:

I showed the mother of a young boy who was autistic how to com- municate with pictures. The next day, she told me, "This morning as I was changing him, I thought I'd download to him what we were going to do. We were going to get dressed and go for a walk. I downloaded the whole morning to him. He just lay there, and then he said, "Shoes?" So, we put on his shoes and then he said, "Walk?"

If you're going to communicate with a kid who is autistic, you have to download the whole shooting match to them. You don't lay it out point by point by point: "Do this, do this, do this, do this." You give them the whole routine, and they can pick that up. They're so fast! But instead of speeding up to where they function, we try to slow them down to live in our reality. That's a mistake we make. Their reality is much faster.

Dain:
Most kids don't have resistance to very much. They're willing to go with the flow, and unlike you, they don't have a time schedule to keep, they don't have to go make money and they're not worried about their pension. They say, "Yeah, Mom, I'll do whatever you want." All you have to do is share it with them.

If there is something your child is in resistance to, you'll know it when you go to give him or her a picture, because the energy will stop right there. It will be, "Uh, this part about you taking me to the dentist. I'm not so sure about that, Mama." You'll know when the resistance starts because you'll feel the energy stop.

Gary:
A mother told us that she downloaded information to her son about going to an appointment with a holistic health practitioner which was going to involve the practitioner touching the boy's spine. The boy objects to being touched, so the mother's aim was make the appointment as smooth and easy as possible.

When she first downloaded information to him about the appointment, he wasn't keen on the idea, so she tried again and sent him a bigger, more complete picture of what was going to happen, and he was all right about going.

On the way home from the appointment, the mother asked him, "How was it?"

The boy said, "Oh, it was good."

The mother asked, "He touched you, didn't he? How did you feel about that?" and the boy replied, "It was nice."

Dain:

Start downloading small bits of information to your kids when they are little, then continue expanding it as they get older. At some point, they'll start downloading to you as well. When that begins to happen, you'll have a connection and a communion with them that will be so extraordinary they won't have to rebel against you in order to have a sense of themselves. And if your kids are already older, know that it's never too late to begin.

Pretty soon your kids will be putting pictures in your head of what they want, and you'll receive them. It happens a little bit at a time. You have to keep practicing. It's like developing a muscle or training to run a five-kilometer race. The first time you try it, you might only be able to run five blocks. You've got to keep doing it.

Gary:

When you start the process of giving them pictures, they'll also start putting pictures in your head. You'll find yourself going to the kitchen to get something for them and you'll stop and ask yourself, "What am I doing? Why am I picking the applesauce?" You won't even know why you're doing it because they didn't ask for the applesauce out loud.

Do your kids ever ignore you when you call for them to come home? When they ignore you, try calling them with your head instead of your voice and see what happens. When you want them to come home, send them a picture of running home really fast. After a while, they'll get the picture and they'll say, "I've got to go home now." All kids have the ability to do this, but we train it out of them by screaming and yelling at them. You've also got to be willing to take the odd step of realizing that you, as well as they, are telepathic.

When Dain and I were doing an X-Men class in Australia, a husband and wife came who had three autistic children. They told me it was a nightmare getting them ready for school in the morning. The kids just wouldn't do what they needed to do to get ready, and they never got to school on time. One kid didn't like to eat, and they fought him to get him to eat breakfast. Another kid would never get into his clothes before he got in the car and even then he didn't want to put them on. He wanted to stay in his pajamas all day long. The third kid just dawdled and was never ready to go.

I said, "You need to give them the schedule for the day in your head, all at once. Just send them a picture of what they're going to have to do for the entire day."

They said, "Okay, we'll try it."

They came back the next night for the class, and they said, "What an amazing day. The kids were up, dressed, fed, and in the car before we were. And at the end of the day, when we usually had to go search them out and chase them down, they were standing on the curb waiting for us. We've never had a day like that. And at dinner, our kid who doesn't like to eat, ate!"

I said, "Yeah, you just have to give them the whole shooting match in one fell swoop." This is the only way these kids perceive. They don't get it when you tell them, "We're going to do this, and then we're going to do this." That is not their reality. Everything happens now for them, so you have to give them a picture of the entire day, and suddenly you'll have kids who are on schedule, doing what they need to do, and doing it the way you need them to do it.

8

PICKING UP OTHER PEOPLE'S THOUGHTS, FEELINGS, AND EMOTIONS

What if you are far more aware than you give yourself credit for?
~ Gary Douglas

Gary:

In the psychological community, Obsessive Compulsive Disorder (OCD) is defined as an anxiety disorder in which the person has unwanted and repeated thoughts, feelings, ideas, sensations (called obsessions) or behaviors that make him or her feel driven to do certain things (called compulsions). It is believed that the person carries out the behaviors to get rid of the obsessive thoughts, but the behavior only provides temporary relief. Not performing the obsessive rituals can cause great anxiety.

There seems to be some truth to these observations, but in our work with people who have OCD, we have discovered something interesting. The thoughts, feelings, and emotions these people have are not actually theirs. They're picking up the thoughts, feelings, and emotions as well as the sex and no sex of everyone else within eight to 8,000 miles around them.

You're probably pretty clear about what thoughts, feelings, and emotions are, but you may not be familiar with the idea of sex and no sex. When we say *sex* and *no sex,* we're not referring to copulation. We chose these words as they bring up the energy of receiving and not receiving better than anything else we've found. People use their points of view about sex and no sex as a way of limiting their receiving. Sex and no sex are exclusionary universes—either/or universes—where you either make your presence known (sex) to the exclusion of everyone else, or you hide your presence (no sex) so that you cannot be seen. In either case, given the focus on yourself, you don't allow yourself to receive from anyone or anything.

Dain:

Imagine picking up every thought, feeling, and emotion, sex and no sex from everybody within an eight-mile radius. Would that give you lots of feelings, thoughts, and emotions? Yeah!

Gary:

Would that tend to overload your system? Yeah! And that's how it feels to people who have OCD.

Dain:

When the system is overloaded like that, doing an action repetitively, like putting something in place or washing your hands, offers some relief. It's the one time you are focused enough on one thing to be able to shut out the awareness of all the information that's coming at you.

Gary:

OCD is called a condition or a disability; however, we consider this kind of awareness an *ability.*

I worked with an eight-year-old girl whose parents were going to put her in special school. She was compulsive beyond belief. She would repeatedly wash her hands and say, "I'm sorry, I'm sorry, I'm sorry." We worked together for two hours, and at the end of two hours, I told the mother that the girl was psychic and picked up information from eighty miles in all directions.

The mother said, "Yeah, right."

About three weeks later, the mother called me and said, "Do you remember when you said that my daughter was psychic beyond belief and she could pick up the feelings, thoughts, and emotions from people all around her? I thought you were full of crap."

This is the most common sentence I hear in my work. She said, "I didn't believe you when you said she could pick up other people's thoughts, but yesterday I was sitting in the car with her. I was thinking how much I loved her, and she turned to me and said, 'I love you too, Mommy.' She heard what I was thinking just like it had been said."

Have you ever had the experience of hearing something and responding to it and then seeing people drop their mouth open and say "Oh!"? You heard it and responded to it—but they didn't say it; they *thought* it. Kids with OCD have these capacities, and so do you.

Eventually, I had to work with this little girl again, because she was besieged by thoughts of having sex with women. I said to her, "Close your eyes and tell me where that energy is coming from."

She closed her eyes and pointed to a garage apartment that was next door.

I asked her father, "Who lives there?"

He said, "A friend of mine."

I said, "Would you please go over there and ask him if he is watching porn?"

It turned out the guy was watching porn for a good portion of his day, and this little girl was picking up his thoughts about having sex with women and thinking there was something dirty about her.

Tool: What Perception Are You Having?

The number one tool you must use with somebody who has OCD is: What perception are you having?

You don't ask, "What emotion, thought, or feeling are you having?" because that makes it *theirs*—and it isn't. It's something they *perceive*.

Dain:

Do you see the difference between *perceiving* something and *feeling* it? If you say, "I feel sad," you have just made yourself sad—even if you weren't. If you *feel* something, you own it, and you are then whatever you have decided you feel.

"I perceive sadness" is a completely different thing. It says, "I am aware of sadness." It's not necessarily something you are being.

Gary:

I perceive so much in my body and everything that is going on in everybody else's body, all at the same time. The only way I can function is if I ask questions about the awareness I'm getting. If I said, "I have this feeling, this feeling, and this feeling," I would be dead meat. I wouldn't be able to walk and talk if I *had* all the stuff I perceive. Knowing that I can *perceive* it or *have the awareness of it* without making it mine creates an amazing difference.

People with ADD, ADHD, and autism also have an exceptional ability to perceive others' feelings, thoughts, and emotions.

Anne:

I was working with the mother of a nine-year-old boy who has been diagnosed with ADHD. He also has many undiagnosed autistic traits. The mom works from home periodically. One day when she was working at home, her son was home as well because there was a teachers' in-service training at his school. The boy was in his bedroom on the second floor of the house, and the mother was in her office on the first floor, where she was engaged in a live meeting on her computer. As the meeting progressed, she was becoming increasingly angry at some of her colleagues.

She told me that she was not speaking or making any sounds. She was not even moving her chair or shuffling papers on her desk. Her son came downstairs, looked at her and asked, "Mom, are you okay?"

She acknowledged that she was angry about stuff at work, not at him, and he said, "Okay, Mom. Just checking! I didn't know if I had done something wrong."

How awesome that he was able to perceive her anger, ask her a question, and not take ownership of it! He knew he hadn't caused her anger, and he did not "feel" her anger either, by becoming angry himself. He simply perceived it.

ADHD and Disruptive Behavior

Gary:

Sometimes a child's ability to perceive others' thoughts, feelings, and emotions can result in what's referred to as disruptive behavior.

I talked with a woman whose daughter was diagnosed with ADHD. When the girl was with her mother, she generally was doing alright. Occasionally, she would have an outburst. When she was with her father and stepmother, she was in a constant state of outburst, and they eventually sent her to boarding school and put her on medication because of it.

The girl was returning to live with her mother, who wanted to know the best way to assist her daughter.

Dain:

People with ADHD have a propensity to pick up the angst and the worry of people around them, and they often have a parent or a spouse who is a worrier.

Gary:

I said to the mother, "She may be acting out because of the situation between her stepmother and father. She may be aware of some discomfort in their universe, but she may not know how to deal with it. Maybe she is trying to deflect from their problems."

The mother said, "All of the above."

I asked, "Will you please claim, own, acknowledge, and recognize that the kid's biggest problem is that she is more aware than her father and stepmother are even willing to consider?"

You've got to remember that kids pick up your feelings, thoughts, and emotions. If you're upset, worried, or concerned about something or if you think there's going to be a problem or that something is going to be difficult, guess what? Kids will pick that up and say, "Oh, this is going to be difficult." You've got to get clear that these kids are far more aware than you give them credit for.

Parents often assume kids shut things out. On the contrary, they're receiving too much information, and they don't know what to do with all of it. Be willing to let go of your stuff so your child doesn't have to have a problem with what's going on in your universe.

Anne:

Kids definitely pick up on their parents' thoughts, feelings, and emotions about them. In an attempt to connect with their parents or to have a loving relationship with their parents, they will do what they can to match those thoughts, feelings, and emotions. I worked with a mom who was constantly at odds with her eight-year-old adopted daughter. She said her daughter did fairly well in school; it was only with her that there were problems and angry outbursts.

She told me her daughter had been placed with her and her husband when the girl was two years old. She had been found by the police, living in a car with her father, who was a drug addict and who died soon thereafter. The mom said, "At two years old, my daughter was 'feral.' She was utterly wild. I thought, given the deprivation and neglect she had experienced, that she would have all kinds of problems, and I set out to fix them for her. I guess I saw her as a problem I needed to fix."

I asked her if she was a good problem solver, and she said she was.

Then I asked, "What if there's nothing wrong with your daughter? What if, by acting out all the time with you, she is helping you to do a good job and be a good mom by allowing you to fix all the problems she presents you with? What if so much of what she's doing is to show you how much she loves you? I wonder what could change if she was no longer your problem."

Tears fell down the woman's face, then she laughed and said, "That's the first thing that anyone has ever said that makes sense to me!" When I saw her the following week, she told me that her daughter's outbursts had all but disappeared. She said that when she stopped thinking that her daughter was a problem that needed to be fixed, there was an energetic shift that occurred between the two of them. For the first time, they had cuddled and snuggled on the couch after the younger siblings had gone to bed, and it had been wonderful. She told me, "It's all so new. I never thought we would be able to spend that kind of time together...ever!"

Tool: Who Does It Belong To?

Gary:

What if you and your body were like a giant radio antenna that picked up thoughts, feelings, and emotions from people all around you? What if 99.9% of every thought, feeling, and emotion you perceived did not belong to you? Guess what? You, just like the kids we're talking about, are constantly picking up thoughts, feelings, and emotions that belong to other people.

Here is a tool you can use when you perceive a feeling, thought, or emotion. You can also teach it to your kids. Ask the question: Who does this belong to?

Do this right now: Get a thought, feeling, or emotion you've had in the past few days or that you're having right now, and ask, "Who does this belong to?"

When you ask that question, does the thought, feeling, or emotion get lighter or go away? Does it get heavier? Or does it stay the same?

If it went away, it's not yours. It was an awareness of someone else's thoughts, feelings, and emotions.

If it got lighter but didn't completely go away, you can return it to sender. You don't even have to know who the sender was. Just say, "Return to sender."

If it got heavier or stayed the same, you have bought that the thought, feeling, or emotion belongs to you. In that case, you can "unbuy" it and return it to sender.

Anne:

A ten-year-old boy who was in the gifted and talented program at a local elementary school struggled with aggressive outbursts toward other kids in his school. He was so quick and so aware—and was flooded by his perceptions of everyone else's thoughts, feelings, and emotions, which he took on as if they were his own. He had been suspended multiple times and truly believed that there was something wrong with him. After one suspension, his dad brought him to my office and we began to work together.

In our sessions, he typically chose to play with Legos and as he created, we talked. One day he said he wished he could stop himself from being aggressive, yet when I offered tools like "Who does that belong to?" he would roll his eyes and shrug his shoulders.

Even so, over time the suspensions decreased in frequency, and he was able to make some friends. That summer, he participated in a "Being Seen and Being Heard" workshop I facilitated. One day he got on stage, and instead of singing like most of the other kids, he chose to talk to the audience. He introduced himself and told everyone that he had gone for several weeks without an outburst, and in fact, had been complimented for being a leader by the staff at the camp he was attending (from which he had been kicked out the previous summer). He then turned to me and said, "You know that 'Who does that belong to' question? It actually works!" He then spoke directly to the audience and explained how it worked and how he had used it to his advantage.

Tool: Who Are You Doing This For?

Gary:

Many kids who have abilities like ADD, ADHD, OCD, and autism pick up the feelings and thoughts of people who think badly of themselves. In truth, somewhere inside themselves, they know they're more able than other people, and they try to take on other people's feelings and thoughts so those people won't feel so bad about themselves. Unfortunately this doesn't work, because you can't take anything away from other people unless they want you to.

Dain:

Most people are not willing to let their bad feelings go, so if you take away their bad feelings, they just make more. And then you try to take those away too. You feel heavier and they make more bad feelings. You take more; they make more. You take more; they make more.

If you perceive that a child is acting out other people's emotions, you can ask: Who are you doing this for? For example, if someone with ADHD says, "I am feeling anxious" or "I am having anxiety," you can ask, "Who are you doing this for?" They will probably realize they are being anxious for someone else."

Gary:

People who are considered disabled have so much more awareness about what's going on than we believe. Many kids are emotionally handicapped simply because they take in too much of the emotion around them. They don't discriminate about what belongs to them and we don't teach them that stuff doesn't belong to them.

Start out by asking your kids these questions and teaching them these tools, and they will begin to use them on their own when their systems get overloaded with information that belongs to other people. These tools take them out of thinking their perception is a feeling they are having.

I love working with kids. They pick up the tools instantaneously and use them right away in all aspects of their life. We allow kids to come to any Access Consciousness class for free until they are sixteen years old. We have a lot of kids who started coming to our classes when they were tiny little guys, and they do all kinds of great things.

Even kids who are very young can learn to use these tools. A little girl in Queensland, Australia was two years old when she came to her first Access Consciousness class. She now knows and uses lots of Access Consciousness tools. One day her mother was having an emotional upset, and the little girl asked, "Mummy, who does that belong to?" and told her to return it to sender.

Mom laughed—and returned it to sender.

9

WORKING WITH KIDS WHO HAVE SPHERICAL AWARENESS

The difference between you and these kids is that you have defined the past as something that has already happened, you see the future as a mystery, and then you have your present, which you think of as a pain in the arse. They don't make that distinction.

~ Gary Douglas

Gary:

Many people with autism have no discriminating factor. This is also true of some people with ADD and ADHD. Their awareness isn't linear the way ours is; they have spherical awareness. Their receivers are on, they are getting 300 channels of television at the same time, and they aren't able to discriminate between one channel and another. And there's no volume control. They receive all that information nonstop and they also simultaneously tap into all their past and future lives. There is no baffle on the information they get.

When they have that much information coming in, they don't know what to do with it, and they either shut down or become dysfunctional in some way.

Dain:

They are trying to put order into something that truly has no order.

Anne:

I recently watched a documentary film about Temple Grandin, an extraordinary, high-functioning woman who has autism. In the film, Grandin describes the way she takes in information, and she tells about a time a high school teacher asked her about shoes. As if to show what was going on in Grandin's mind, the screen explodes with hundreds of pictures of shoes of all kinds and Grandin talking as fast as she can, attempting to describe each and every shoe that came to mind, past, present and future, all jumbled together. She said she looked for patterns in the midst of all that information and tried so hard to describe it in ways that made sense to her teacher, which was really a difficult task.

Gary:

That's exactly where so many of these kids function from. You ask a question, and they pick it up from a totally different place, and you're left going "What?" But if you hang in there with the communication, they will eventually bring it around so the snake's head bites its tail; suddenly everything they are saying connects with the question you asked.

These kids don't have the construct of past, present, and future the way we do; that's not the way they function. They don't think of things in terms of day-to-day, Monday, Tuesday, Wednesday. That construct doesn't have any meaning for them. I think it's more like, "I see all this week, all last week, and all the other weeks. And how come any of this matters to you guys?"

It's much closer to an animal's point of view. The horse doesn't say, "Okay, I have to carry this stupid rider around for the next twenty years before I can be out to pasture." It just says, "Oh, I'm going to do this? I'm going to do that? Okay, fine."

We create meaning based on time, but they don't see the significance of time in the way we do. We say things like "We've been together twenty years" or "This happened 200 years ago." They ask, "Why does this matter? Why are you making this important? I don't get it." If you looked at your life from the point of view that you could live for 1,000 years, what would you make important about today? Would it be the fact that you're going to party tonight?

It is the same with money. Our point of view is that kids have to learn to put on their clothes, go out in the world, work, and earn money. They say, "Huh? Why? What's important about that? The amount of money you have today is important based on what?" They don't have those concepts.

So, we try to linearize things for them. We try to teach them to discriminate one channel from another, which is not a characteristic or a capacity they have. Instead of trying to get them to linearize things, we need to give them tools they can use to work with their spherical awareness.

Tool: Is This Past, Present, or Future?

It often helps these kids when you ask whether something is past, present, or future. When someone functions in the simultaneity of time, space, dimensions, and realities, everything is *now*. What happened four trillion years ago is right now. They are also in the future, doing the future as well. If you begin to help them delineate whether something is past, present, or future, they can start to create some order in their universe. Currently they do not have a reference point for that.

Kids who have the simultaneous capacities we're talking about can see what's going to happen in the future, and for many of them, it's frightening. They can see the limitations that are being created every day, because their universe changes moment by moment, every ten seconds. They can see that when you make *that* choice, *this* is going to happen.

Is that an ability? Yes, it is an ability. If we all had that ability, would we have made the mistakes we have made on this planet? If you knew that you were going to be in an accident if you drove your car down a certain street, would you go down that street or would you take a different route? These kids can see that going down that street isn't going to work—but they can't make you see it. Can you imagine the distress and frustration this creates for them?

In the same way, a lot of these kids pick up all the sorrow in the world. The majority of people on this planet run on sadness, grief, and anger as though that's the truth of life, and many of these kids are overwhelmed by these feelings. They perceive them with such intensity because they have no regulators on it.

We can say, "Oh, this sadness isn't mine. I picked it up from this person" or "I'm sad because this event happened." For them, there is no event connected to the sadness; it simply exists—and it is everywhere. It is pervasive in their world.

Most kids with autism seem to live in their own private universe. They are so overloaded with sensory input that they respond to it by creating a private universe to live in.

We heard about a little girl who was having psychotic episodes and building bomb shelters two days before 9/11. She was picking up information about the terrorist attack before it happened. She ended up in a hospital, drugged out of her mind, and that's a difficulty, because you cannot drug people out of awareness. It doesn't work. When we don't acknowledge people's abilities and their capacities, we make them more agitated, not less. And they are not disabled; they are very aware—in a different way than we are.

Have you ever been around somebody who is really angry and not expressing it? You can feel all that energy. It's totally real to you, but when you mention it to them, they might say, "What are you talking about? Nothing's wrong." You know something's wrong, and they're denying it. That's what it's like for autistic kids. They perceive it all, but no one acknowledges what they perceive. Their world seems abusive. They are being hit with sticks and stones. It's very difficult and uncomfortable for them. Acknowledging what's happening and asking, "Is this past, present, or future?" begins to unlock this situation for them.

10

BEING IN NATURE, CONNECTING WITH ANIMALS, PLAYING, AND EXPLORING THE WORLD

Animals have tremendous gifts they can give to us if we're willing to receive them. Horses, in particular, want to take care of us. Have you ever noticed that sometimes after you ride a horse you feel really expanded, joyful, and happy? Why does that occur? It's because you've been willing to receive from the horse.

- Gary Douglas

Gary:

I talked with a parent who asked, "Is it possible that we react to kids with ADD and other conditions as though there is something wrong with them because we're accustomed to the traditional ways of raising of children, where we say, 'Sit down and shut up. Eat when you're told. Go to bed when it's your bedtime'?"

This person's perception was that an evolution of the species has been going on for some time, and this includes an evolution in the awareness of children. There's a generation coming through who are more aware and more active, and people are saying, "There is something wrong with this generation of kids. There must be something we need to do, because disciplining them isn't working." This kind of discussion has been going on for many years.

Part of what's going on is that the perception of how to raise a child has shifted 180 degrees in recent times. In many respects, we've taken childhood away from children. Kids are given hours of homework to do, even when they're in kindergarten. Their lives are highly organized and tightly scheduled. They have little time to play in unstructured ways, to be in nature, or to explore their world. When does a kid get to be a kid? They should be able to go outside and play, have a good time, and run around.

Anne:

Kids are so aware of the benefits of play. They are demanding to play, and they are letting us know how silly it is not to. Play serves many functions in a developing child. It is through play that a child's verbal language, physical, psychological, social, and cognitive/intellectual skills are developed. For young children whose verbal skills do not allow them to express themselves as ours do, play is a primary form of communication. It is through their play that they share with us their inner world. It is by their invitation to us to play with them that we are afforded a glimpse of what their world looks like and feels like to them. Garry Landreth, one of the first child therapists to recognize the healing potential of bringing play into the therapy room, said, "Toys are words and play is language."

A four-and-half-year-old girl with a diagnosis of Separation Anxiety Disorder was referred to me by her pediatrician. According to her mom, when it was time to go to school, the girl would wail and sob and cling to her. Mom was exhausted, as was her daughter, as was the staff at her preschool program. The girl was only attending school four half-days (instead of five full days) per week, and Mom was in despair. School staff reported that the girl sobbed and cried for a good portion of the mornings, and that she "refused to participate in classroom activities, kept to herself, made little eye contact, and did not respond to staff or other children."

In my initial meetings with Mom, she described everything she had tried to assist her daughter, as well as all the suggestions she received from the school staff, relatives, and other parents, most of which were based on how wrong the girl's behavior was—none of which worked. I then met with her daughter.

She was a lovely girl, bright-eyed, curious, and on the quiet side. She invited me into her play within a couple of sessions. I did not find her to be as she had been described to me at all. I asked her some questions as we played with dolls and the doll house.

Me: Could you tell me what it is about school that you so dislike?

The girl: No toys!

Me: No toys?! (She was attending an alternative program that did in fact have toys, but there was no free play. The toys were to be played with in a certain way, in a certain place, at a certain time.)

The girl: No toys!

Me: What's it like to be in a school with no toys?

The girl: *Not fun!*

Me: Hmm…

And that was it!

Ten days later, her mom came back to see me by herself. She told me that on the day following our session, her daughter got herself up, dressed herself, and was eager to go to school. When they arrived at school, she said goodbye to her mom with no tears. That afternoon, she asked her mom if she could go to school all day, which she did, after the holidays that were coming up.

What if it was my simple acknowledgement that it *is* silly not to be able to play in school the way we were playing in the play therapy room was all the girl required to choose a different way of being with school?

Dain:

Kids need time to explore their world and see what it's like. They need to learn everything they can learn on their own, not just from a mental perspective but from an energetic point of view.

Anne:

A study conducted at the University of Illinois in 2011 found that kids diagnosed with ADHD have milder symptoms if they play outdoors, in green grassy spaces and parks daily, or at least several days a week.

Gary:

A friend of ours has a farm, and she invites kids with autism, OCD, ADD and ADHD to go there to spend some time in nature with the animals. She said that after a few days of being there, the kids all settle down. There is a sense of peace there that they don't get in the city.

In part, that's because many of them hear the electrical wires humming in the city. They're aware of the vibration that electricity creates. It's not a wrongness; it's an ability to perceive the vibration of the electric wires, which is everywhere in a city. The kids pick it up, but they have no reference point for what they're hearing, and they don't know what to do with it. When they go out away from the city, the buzz goes away.

The other thing that contributes to their sense of peace is contact with the animals. We know a lady in the U.S. who has been working with autistic kids and horses, and she said it's amazing how often kids who are out of control—the ones who scream, yell, and kick—

become calm when they ride. She said as soon as they get off the horse, they lie down on the ground and take a nap. The horse creates a sense of calm in the kids because it picks up on their wavelength. It telepathically understands what the kids are trying to say.

There are many horses with healing abilities that will take care of children. They will create a communion with kids in a very dynamic way. The horse always knows which kid it wants. It doesn't necessarily like all kids, and it won't have anything to do with the ones it doesn't like, but if it makes a connection with a kid, they can have an amazing relationship.

This kind of connection and communion also happens between kids and other kinds of animals. Dogs, especially, like having a job, and many of them have great healing abilities. Our friend, Suzy, who is a dog whisperer of magnitude, told us about a dog she worked with. The dog's owner was a woman whose child had autism. The woman was overwhelmed by taking care of her child, and she decided she couldn't deal with the dog and the child, so she gave the dog away.

When the dog got to his new home, he started ripping up the carpet. At that point, Suzy was called in to communicate with him, and it turned out that the dog knew he was beneficial to the autistic child and he wanted to go back to be with him—but the original owner wouldn't allow that to occur. It was a shame, because the dog clearly had abilities and wanted to make a contribution to the child.

Animals are like people. They have different abilities. It's a tremendous gift for all kids, especially kids with autism, to have an animal in their life. Horses, in particular, are great because they communicate telepathically. They are so grateful when somebody receives their communication that they will nurture that person in a special way.

11

THE ZONE

These kids don't see the world the same way we do.
We won't see through their eyes, which is our mistake. It's our
wrongness, not theirs. We need to see what they see rather than try to
get them to see things our way.
– Gary Douglas

Gary:

Years ago, I used to train horses, and after I started doing Access Consciousness, I began to look for better ways to create a sense of communion and connection with the horses I worked with. In the course of doing this, I discovered that each horse has a zone in which everything is peaceful. In the zone, there is a sense of communion, connection, and knowing. I found when I worked with horses that if I created a zone that matched the horse's zone, it was a place where we could both connect.

Dain says it helps him to think about the zone in terms of space.

Dain:

This exercise might allow you to have more awareness of what the zone is.

> Close your eyes. Reach out with your awareness and touch the eight corners of the room you're in. Just expand your awareness

out. Now expand your awareness out even further, so that you're out ten miles in all directions. Now a hundred. Now five hundred. Now a thousand.

Gary:

Most of us tend to walk around with very little awareness of the space around us. Sometimes our space is the size of our brain. It's important to be aware of this, because when we work with animals, we need to adjust our space to the amount of space the animal is comfortable with. All animals have a sense of awareness of space and a level at which they feel comfortable and secure. Have you ever had a dog or cat that liked to be in the house all the time and hated to go outside? The only area it was willing to occupy was the house. Or have you had an animal that only wanted to be outdoors? I've had cats that insisted on being outside. They'd look up at the sky and all around them and check everything out. When you're with an animal like that, you have to have the same kind of awareness it has in order for it to be in communion and connection with you.

I have a stallion at a ranch near Santa Barbara, and in order to ride him, my space has to be about eighteen miles out in all directions. A stallion's job is to protect the herd, so if you're going to ride one, you need to occupy the same amount of space that it needs to occupy in order for it to feel safe and calm. If I close the space down when I ride my stallion, he goes frantic. He feels like he's being trapped. But if I extend my awareness out far enough, I can ride him into a herd of other horses and he walks along like a gelding. He's calm and comfortable because I perceive everything that he perceives, and he feels safe.

At one of our animal workshops, we worked with a dog that was found as a puppy in the wild, and even after living with people for many years, she was still very shy. She didn't trust people and wouldn't go up to them. If a stranger walked up to her, she would start to tremble. We ran a number of Access Consciousness processes on her, but she didn't begin to truly relax until I asked the dog's owner to feel how far out the dog's zone went and to expand his awareness out to all the things his dog was aware of. The dog was paying attention to all the smells, sights, sounds, and energies for miles around.

We worked with the dog's owner until he got the idea of expanding into the dog's space, rather than trying to contract the dog into his space. He finally expanded into the dog's space and almost immediately, the dog got calmer and her eyes became softer. That was the amount of space she needed to achieve the zone of quietude, relax, and connect more fully with the world.

I told the owner, "It's important not to ask too much of a dog like this. Ask a little bit, and when the dog gives it, ask just a little bit more, and it will give you that. Rather than trying to get your dog to be with people, accept whatever it gives as friendliness, thank it, reward it for that, and acknowledge its space and its zone continuously. The more you do that, the more friendly and ease-filled the dog will be."

People have a zone too. There is a zone they occupy that is natural to them. This is the space in which they feel a sense of calm and safety and have the capacity to connect.

Let's say you have a child who is overwhelmed by all the information he is receiving.

He doesn't have the ability to limit the information that's coming in. He's picking up everything that's going on, including all the thoughts, feelings, and emotions of everyone around him. It's all there in his universe; there is no division between what's right and what's wrong, what's good and what's bad, what's now and what's past, what's his and what's not.

You can create the zone for him. When you create the zone for kids, you establish a place where connection and communion can exist, and they will begin to understand that they can create the zone for themselves.

Dain:

Initially it's something you do for them. You take their energy and expand it into the zone. With a very young child, you can say, "Here you go, honey," and just expand the space he occupies.

Gary:

All of a sudden, he'll look around, and you'll know you've done it.

You can also create the zone for kids when they are in challenging situations. For example, I talked with a teacher about a student who became very unsettled when he was in a school assembly, surrounded by other kids. He would begin to make a lot of distracting noises.

I said, "If you can create the zone for him, he will start to feel the energy of it, and it will get him more calm in his body. You just have to pull the space out that so he doesn't contract under those circumstances. Eventually, he will recognize that he can expand and not be over-stimulated."

You have to work at creating a sense of space for these kids, because when things come at them, they feel so impacted. It's like somebody is continuously hitting them upside the head. They say, "I can't deal with this" and they try to check out—except there's no real way for somebody with so much awareness to check out.

Keep creating that space, and they will begin to realize that there is a way for them to create it too. Once they feel you do it, they'll ask, "Hey, what did Mom or Dad just do? What did the teacher just do? Oh, I can do that."

Dain and I talked with a parent whose kids couldn't handle wearing clothing for long periods of time. The kids always wanted to get naked. It was as if they were overloaded and confined by the sensory input they were receiving, including the feeling of the clothes they were wearing—not to mention the thoughts they were picking up from the people around them. We suggested that the parent expand the kids' zone.

It is also helpful when you expand the zone for yourself. When you do this, the thoughts, feelings, and emotions you're picking up won't impact you the same way, and this calms and soothes your child.

You can create that space, that zone in which they feel, "Oh, I've got more space." If you start doing this, it will help them tremendously.

Anne:

Before I met Gary and Dain, I did not realize that I was expanding the zone of the kids I worked with. I could not explain clearly how it was that kids who had disliked other therapists were able to connect with me so quickly and make so many gains. However, now it makes perfect sense to me.

I create the zone for kids—and for their parents—and it provides them with a space where there is peace and calm. They can relax. They are able to let down their guard and take a look at the elements in their lives and relationships that brought them to see me in the first place. Creating the zone for them is a way of letting them be without judging them and of asking questions so that they can become more aware of what they are creating and what other choices they could make.

One of the ways I try to create the zone for kids is by totally receiving them. When I first meet them, it's as if I open up all the pores in my body. I look at them and say, "Hi!" It might seem like a simple greeting, but it's so much more than that. It's the energy of "I'm so glad our paths are crossing. You are awesome just the way you are. Whatever you say or do is fine with me. And I will give you whatever space you require to have what you would like to have. You are welcome to join me in my space." When I do this, their response, almost always, is to relax, and often they then invite me into their space.

I have been asked how I work with kids who don't want to be in the play therapy room with me. I never force kids to come into the room with me if they don't want to. What I do is expand their zone, and with rare exceptions, they always choose to come into the room. The zone is the place we connect.

Oftentimes a kid's zone collapses when he or she feels criticized, invalidated, or "wrong." When this occurs, it often helps kids expand their zones if I ask questions that assist them to see the truth of themselves.

A ten-year-old girl who is brilliant, high functioning, and easily agitated recently came to see me again after a break of three years. She was scowling at me and her mom, unhappy about being back in my office. When I asked her why she had come back, she said, "My mom thinks there's something wrong with my brain."

I asked Mom if she thought there was something wrong with her daughter's brain.

Mom replied, "No, not at all!"

The girl looked at me, and without using any words, said, "Not true!"

I asked her, "Would you like to know where I am with all that?"

She nodded *yes*.

I said, "I don't think there is anything wrong with you. In fact, I think you are an amazingly talented girl with capacities that other people don't have. Can I ask you a couple of questions?"

She nodded *yes.*

"Does your mind move quicker than other people's?"

She nodded *yes.*

"Do you know what other people are thinking and feeling, even when they don't tell you with their words?"

She nodded *yes.*

"When somebody says or does something, can you tell how it's going to turn out, even before it happens?"

She nodded *yes.*

"Sometimes do you get frustrated or mad when people don't or can't keep up with you?"

She nodded *yes.*

"What if there was really nothing wrong with you? What if you could learn some tools so it was easier for you to be seen and heard and to have everything you would like to have in your life?"

Her body lightened up, she started to smile, then tried to stop herself—but couldn't— before a giggle came out.

"Yes!" her mom said, "That's what I was trying to say! I just didn't know how."

Kids love being given permission to be in their zone. When they sense they have that permission, they become willing to learn tools they can use to be seen and heard so they can get along in the outside world with more ease and peace. I ask them if they can "hold the space of who and where they are," then while holding that space and staying in their zone, if they can step into other people's worlds in order to give those people what they require.

Gary:

We can all function in this way all the time. Instead we tend to contract our lives into a small space, as though that's really all we have to worry about. When we do that, we create our worry space. But what about our awareness space? If we functioned with an expansive point of view, an awareness space, we wouldn't run into problems. It's definitely the space we want to function from.

~ 12 ~

WHEN KIDS SEEM FAR AWAY

*Because of autism, I was constantly thinking about what I saw
in such extreme detail that it seemed like I wasn't thinking at all.
- Twelve-year-old boy with autism*

Anne:

Sometimes kids become so wrapped up in what they are doing that
it seems as if they disappear. We use phrases like "in another world"
or "wrapped up in their own world" to describe them.

When parents try to get their attention, oftentimes they are met
with silence. To some, it appears as if their child did not even hear
them. It would be easy to view this as a sign of disrespect, opposi-
tion, or defiance. What if it's not? What if the kids are so tuned in
to what they are doing that their parent's voice doesn't even register
with them? Many kids just need some time to disconnect from what
they are engaged in, especially if it's fun, before they can move on
to something that is not so fun, like going to school or coming to
the dinner table. If we impatiently *demand* that they leave where
they are and come back into this reality *now*, things usually don't go
so well. They don't want to leave that quickly, and they push back
hard, either by trying to block us out or by exploding. And then we
get upset.

What if the demand could be turned into an invitation or a request? And what if the request could be presented in a way that is easier on you, your child, and everyone involved? What if you could approach them in a calm and respectful way, so that they can hear?

Sometimes you can get a child's attention if you simply say, "Hi!" If you are in a rush, though, chances are pretty good your child will remain where she is, but if you can be present with her and tap into where she is, chances are much better that she will be willing to join you where you are.

The parents of a seven-year-old boy who is on the autism spectrum and receiving services in his public school described to me how he loves being by himself and playing with Legos for hours at a time. Everyone else in the family, his parents and three siblings, are outgoing. They love to eat in restaurants, go out to movies, and travel to new places, none of which he likes to do. His mom told me that he was "ruining" family outings because he typically threw such big fits about going out that no one wanted to be with him.

One day when I was meeting with the parents alone, they asked me about all of this. Mom's point of view was that her son needed to act more like the rest of the family and quit being so different. She was angry at him for "controlling" everyone. Her approach with her son tended to be confrontational, which invariably led to outbursts, tears, and despair. Dad was more relaxed about the boy. He tended to be more patient and to have a kinder view of his son's behavior, although he acknowledged that he too was frustrated by the frequent conflicts.

Dad told me that the night before when they had gone out to eat, their son had joined them without incident. He asked Mom whether she had noticed. She said, "Yeah, but it doesn't happen very often."

I asked them what had been different. Dad said that twenty minutes before it was time to leave the house, he had found his son playing with his Legos in the basement and had sat down next to him. He told me, "We just hung out together, and after a while, I reminded him that soon we would be leaving to go eat. He kept on playing. He showed me what he was doing, and I was right there with him. Every so often I reminded him that we would be leaving. Then, when it was time to leave, he said he'd rather stay home, but he put on his shoes and came anyway."

Mom looked at him, paused, and said, "I don't have that kind of time!" to which Dad replied, "But you have time for three-hour tantrums?"

One of the underlying principles of my work with kids and families over the years has been that behavior is a form of communication. I ask parents, "What's your child saying to you when he throws a tantrum? When she cries inconsolably? When he doesn't want to leave the house? When she disappears into her own world?"

What worked about the father's approach? My point of view is that by quietly hanging out with the boy by acknowledging his interests and his preference for staying home without trying to talk him out of it or suggesting that there was something wrong with him, the dad connected with his son energetically. He became an invitation to the boy to join him and the rest of the family in their evening out. What if that was all that was required for them to have a peaceful evening together?

Kids can become so involved in doing things, it's almost as if they are *in* the book or they *become* the book, the game, or the movie, rather than reading the book, watching the movie, or playing the game. Gary suggested the following questions, which I've found to be very effective in getting kids to join me where I am. These questions do, however, have to be asked in a friendly and non-accusative way:

- Where are you?
- Did you just disappear?
- Are you aware that you can stay outside the book and still be aware of everything in the book?

Tool: Expanding Out in All Directions

When I work with kids, especially kids who become so completely involved doing things that they resist being with others, I encourage them to have the awareness they have, and at the same time, to see, listen, and hear right here, right now, which expands their attention out in all directions. When they expand out in all directions, they can be aware of all that they are aware of and still function in this reality with teachers, parents, and other family members in a way that's easy on them and everyone around them.

Here's a way you can teach kids to do this that I learned from Dain and then added to. (It's something you can do yourself as well!)

Get comfortable, either sitting down or lying down. Close your eyes.

Get a sense of your being and your body. Your being is what goes on forever. Some people call it your soul or your spirit. Dr. Seuss says there is no one who is "youer than you."

Then get a sense of your body. Is your body in your being, or is your being in your body? Your body is in your being!

Now, make your being bigger than your body...

Bigger than the room...

Expand out in all directions, up, down, right, left, forward, backward...bigger...

Bigger than your town...

Bigger than your country...

Bigger than the planet...

Bigger...!

Bigger than from here to the Moon...

Bigger than from here to Jupiter...

All the way to the outside edges of the Universe...

There...from that space, is there anything upsetting you? Can you even see an upset?

If you do this exercise with your kids, they will be able to do it by themselves, no matter where they are. From that space, they'll be able to give teachers, parents, other kids, or coaches whatever is required in the moment, without losing themselves.

Again, it's simple. Ask them to expand out and be present. They'll get the hang of this quickly, and they'll see immediately how much easier life can be.

Beware!

If you teach these tools to your kids, they will offer to use them with you.

A mother told me that she and her six- and nine-year-old daughters were in their car, on the highway.

Mom: Oh, I have such a headache!

Nine year old: Mom, who does that belong to?

Mom (laughing because the headache diminished instantly): Oh, not me! Thanks!

Six year old: Mom, do you want me to help make you bigger?

Mom: Sure!

Six year old: Okay, Mom, shut your eyes.

Nine year old: Bad idea. She's driving.

Six year old: Okay, Mom, keep your eyes open and make yourself bigger than the car…bigger than the highway…

How does it get any better than that?

"Expanding Out" is one of my favorite Access Consciousness tools, and I use it often. It creates space instantly in my body that allows me to respond and act differently and in ways that are so much easier on me and on everyone around me!

Tool: Who Are You Being? Where Are You?

My friend Trina is an occupational therapist in the public school system. She says she often uses a variation of the Expanding Out tool. One day she was working with a five-year-old girl who has been diagnosed with autism, among other syndromes. The girl makes little to no eye contact. Frequently, she bangs her head on the floor, cries, screams, and ramps up into noisy, dramatic outbursts.

On these occasions, Trina says the girl's name then asks her, "Who are you being?" Sometimes Trina has to repeat her name and the question several times. Trina has a gentle, soothing way about her, so she does this without being confrontational. When she does this, the girl almost always calms down, and Trina will ask, "Where are you?" At that point, Trina says the girl calms down even more and makes eye contact with her. Trina then asks her, "What if you could stay there and come and play with me here?" When she does that, the girl maintains eye contact and is able to be present and play with her.

My early training emphasized that seeming far away was a sign of disrespect. I knew at the time that it wasn't; I just didn't know what it was. I am so grateful to have these tools to use and pass on. We encourage you to play with these tools. Have fun with them. And let us know what you and your children are able to create together.

13

WHAT IF ADD AND ADHD
WERE ACTUALLY GIFTS?

People with ADD and ADHD are the greatest
multi-taskers in the universe.
~ Dr. Dain Heer

Gary:

In recent years, a huge number of kids have been diagnosed with ADD and ADHD, and doctors often try to put them on drugs such as Ritalin to slow them down. From what I've seen, this is a big mistake. My oldest daughter had ADD and they wanted to put her on Ritalin, so I started doing some research to find out what its long-terms effects are.

Ritalin is a nervous system stimulant and it acts differently on different kids. It makes some kids more impulsive, which may explain why a noticeably large percentage of the boys (and a smaller percentage of the girls) who are put on it engage in criminal behavior as they get older. In some states, the question, "Are you on Ritalin?" has been added to routine police reports involving juveniles. Other kids' nervous systems are overwhelmed by Ritalin, and it makes them into nice, well-behaved zombies.

Anne:

A mother of a boy, now in his twenties, told me that he was diagnosed with ADHD when he was a child. She said, "I fought a family of doctors to keep him away from Ritalin and the low sugar diet. I just knew he was different and a lot more aware than other kids. Today he is on his way to joining the London School of Economics for his master's degree in subjects that are not run-of-the mill stuff. In addition to that, he writes music, film scripts, and short stories, and he is a wonderful, warm, and aware being."

It might be worth asking whether putting your child on medications is actually required, or whether other possibilities are available.

Gary:

Personally, I don't believe any drug is truly good for the body. I figure your body has the ability to adjust itself if you are willing to allow it to, so I tried to discover how I could deal with my daughter's so-called inability to focus. When I started to work with her, I quickly discovered that if she had the television and the radio on at the same time, she could do all her homework in about twenty minutes. Why is that? Because the sensory input levels at which she can receive information are far greater than most of us have.

Kids who have ADD or ADHD try to put their attention on one thing, and before they even get their attention settled on it, their attention has already shifted to another place. And by the time they get focused on the second thing, they have shifted their attention to yet another place. Maybe they will go back to the first thing, maybe not.

You can avoid the frustration of trying to make them focus on one thing if you realize they need a greater degree of sensory input than the average person and allow them to have the input they require to be comfortable.

Parents aren't always comfortable with letting their kids do this. They believe kids are only capable of doing one thing at a time, but this is clearly not the case. A mother asked me, "What do you do with a child who has the ability to do his homework with the TV and radio on but who has a parent that insists he can't do more than one thing at a time?"

I asked, "So, you're not the parent?"

She said, "No, I'm the other parent."

I said, "Say to the other parent, "Hey, I talked with this weird guy the other day and he had an idea for something we could do with our son. Do you want to try it?"

The mother said, "He'll say, 'Since *weird* is the operative word, no.' Isn't there something I can say to him that would make him stop having a fixed point of view?"

I said, "In that case, every time he says, 'No, that can't work' or 'No, I don't want our son to do this,' you can say (in your head), 'Everything he just said, destroy and uncreate it,' which may help undo the solid energy of his refusal to try something new."

Then I said, "You can probably get your son to do his homework before his dad gets home if you say, 'If you'll do your homework immediately after school, I'll let you watch TV and listen to the radio while you do it.'"

Dain:

People with ADD and ADHD are the greatest multi-taskers in the universe. They can listen to the radio, watch the television, and take in the conversation that's going on around them while they are doing their homework. They say, "Oh, I finally have enough to do!" They are always looking for more sensory input.

Gary:

They want more to do, more to do, and more to do, which is why they are considered disruptive in school. They go from one thing to another. It's "Hey, what are you doing?" They want to be involved in everything. Their point of view is "What else can I add to my life? What else can I do? What else can I do?" Kids who have this ability have a great need to do many things. They are the most joyful and productive when they have more to do than they can possibly accomplish.

Anne:

As a multi-tasker of magnitude, one of the greatest gifts I received from Gary and Dain was the realization that it's okay to do more than one thing at a time. My grade school report cards said things like "Doesn't live up to her full potential" and "Doesn't complete her work in a timely manner." I thought there was something wrong with me because my teachers kept saying that I couldn't pay attention, focus, concentrate, or finish things. I remember being told by one of my brothers that he and his wife used to place bets on how long I could stay seated when I went upstairs to study. It was never long before I would get up to find something, get a drink of water, turn on the radio, call a friend, or read a magazine.

Today I function best when I have several projects going on at the same time. How do I know what to pick up? I ask. It's always a simple question, like: What am I meant to be doing? Who am I meant to be talking to? Which project requires my attention now? When I ask these questions, I always seem to know what to do next. I no longer function from the space of feeling wrong for not finishing one thing before starting the next. I'll write, create classes, do laundry, work in the garden, make soup, and talk on the phone—and somehow everything gets done. For me, this is a joyful—and also productive—way to operate. And when I have only one thing to do, it takes me forever to get it done.

Jake

A friend of mine who is a consultant to an elementary school told me about an experience she had with a boy who had ADHD.

She was sent out to a school to work with some students. The first person they wanted her to work with was a boy named Jake. They said, "He is so ADHD! Wait until you see him. He's hyper-hyper-hyper." My friend said, "It was as if every time they said, 'Jake,' they were nominating him as the poster boy for ADHD."

She went into Jake's classroom and introduced herself to his teacher, Miss Smith. As she was talking to Miss Smith, Jake was standing at Miss Smith's side, moving his hands, tapping her on the shoulder and saying, "Miss Smith, Miss Smith, Miss Smith."

Every time he would say her name, Miss Smith would say, "In a minute, Jake; in a minute, Jake." My friend watched Miss Smith's frustration increasing as the two of them tried to continue their conversation. She could see that Miss Smith was about to hit her limit and Jake was going to get blasted, so she turned from Miss Smith and said, "Hey Jake."

He said, "Yep?"

She said, "You know how you can hear thirty-five people at one time?"

He said, "Uh huh."

She said, "Guess what? Miss Smith can't do that; she can only hear one person at a time. Do you think you could honor that, and know there's nothing wrong with you, and there's nothing wrong with Miss Smith?"

Jake said, "Sure," and he stopped.

My friend knew that in his universe, Jake was not interrupting them. He can do a million things at one time, and he didn't have the awareness that other people might not have the ability to operate that way as well. In acknowledging Jake's ability to hear many people at one time rather than reprimanding him for his inability to stand quietly and wait, my friend let Jake know what was needed in this circumstance without blasting him or making him different, disabled, or wrong. In fact, she let him know that he was a pretty cool kid—he just needed to wait until she and Miss Smith finished their conversation—because Miss Smith didn't function the way he did.

14

BEING WITH KIDS WHO HAVE
ADD OR ADHD

*When you step into something different, you open up the space for
that to exist, where before there was no space for it to be.*

~ Dr. Dain Heer

Anne:

In the previous chapter, we talked about ADD and ADHD as a gift
and they certainly can be that. We also recognize that ADD and
ADHD can be a challenge for kids, parents, and teachers, as kids
with ADD and ADHD can seem driven or frantic, and some have a
tendency to erupt. It is easy to become frustrated with them. Sometimes they appear to be so scattered, distracted, and unfocused. Parents and teachers want them to pay attention to something, complete a task, or sit quietly—and their attention goes all over the
place. They want to be involved in everything. It can be downright
exasperating!

A friend who is a member of the special education staff at an elementary school told me the following story about a boy she called
Joey who had been labeled with ADHD. It is one of my favorite
stories, as it illustrates the gift of awareness that is part of ADD and
ADHD—as well the challenges parents and educators face in dealing with kids whose attention seems to be drawn in so many different directions.

My friend had been asked to do an evaluation of Joey, so the two of them went to a quiet place on the school grounds and sat together as she gathered information for the evaluation. She was aware that he was listening to her and was willing to participate in the tasks at hand. However, despite his willingness to engage with her, he would often turn his head to look at something or his eyes would dart in one direction or another.

In a classroom, this could have been interpreted as distractibility or a lack of attention. The teacher might have concluded, "Oh, he's not listening to me." However, my friend knew it was not lack of attention. She could see that he was aware of, and being pulled by, an energy.

She asked him "Hey, what's up? What is that?" to which he replied, "Oh, that's kids walking."As he said that, she became aware of kids walking in the hallway on the other side of the campus. Not many people would have heard it, and she acknowledged his perception. She knew that if she had told him that he was distracted or not paying attention, she would have invalidated him and what he was aware of.

They continued with the evaluation, and a few minutes later, she saw his attention shift away again. She asked, "What's that?" He said, "Kids talking." She said, "Okay," and tuned in. Sure enough, across the schoolyard, kids were talking.

A short while later, his eyes darted towards the sky. She asked, "What's happening?"

He replied, "An airplane." She thought to herself, "Oh, that's interesting. There's no airplane," then a minute later, she heard the plane. He was aware of it before it was audible or visible to her. He had perceived the energy of it coming.

What if the frustration and exasperation you may experience with your child's ADD or ADHD doesn't have to dictate your relationship with your child? What if it doesn't have to define your relationship? What if there is a way to acknowledge and appreciate your child's abilities—even in the midst of his or her scattered or unfocused behavior?

And what if there are some things you can do that will actually assist your child with ADD or ADHD?

ADD and ADHD—What's the Difference?

Prior to 1994, the only difference between ADD and ADHD was the "H," which stands for *hyperactivity*. ADD, or attention deficit disorder, described the symptoms dealing with inattention; ADHD, or attention deficit hyperactivity disorder, described those symptoms as well as hyperactivity and impulsivity. Then, in 1994, ADD was dropped as a diagnosis by the medical community, and ADHD was given three subcategories: 1) predominantly inattentive (the old ADD); 2) predominantly hyperactive and/or impulsive; and 3) the combined type. Although that was the official change, today many people still refer to ADD to describe inattention.

Implants

One of the things Gary and Dain have discovered is that implants are responsible for many of the difficulties connected with ADD and ADHD.

Most people are familiar with the idea of dental implants or breast implants, which are about implanting substances into the physical body. We're not talking about those kinds of implants here, though; we're referring to energetic implants. For example, a song that repeats itself over and over in your head is an implant. When someone like a parent, a teacher, or a friend tells you something is true that really isn't true, and you believe it—or keep replaying it—that's an implant. Something you do by habit, like twisting your hair, is an implant. There is no awareness in it. The song, the false statement, or the habit has been implanted into your universe and it keeps repeating itself over and over again.

Oftentimes implants also include thoughts, feelings, and emotions that have been inserted in your universe. For example, if you were repeatedly told as a child by a parent that you were stupid and you were labeled with a learning disability, you would believe that it was true. The judgment, "You're stupid" would become an implant in your universe.

I have a friend, now in his forties, who is brilliant. He has created a multimillion dollar business, and he is on the cutting edge of his field. He confided in me recently that he spent his secondary education years in special education classrooms because he had been "branded" as learning disabled. His response to the shame and degradation to which he was subjected was to act out, and he gave his parents and teachers a run for their money! He was told he would never be accepted into college because he was slow and not a good learner. It was not true. As I said, he is brilliant. Is he different? Yes! Does he think like others do? No!

Unfortunately, like many X-Men kids, he had no tools he could use to cope with the craziness that was his life, and he spent many years drinking, trying to numb himself to the awareness he had, which just validated the judgment that he was stupid and dumb and that people in his life could never see his brilliance and could not acknowledge what was true. My friend no longer drinks, yet in spite of the success of his business, he still fights the demons of being stupid and not good enough. Sadly, mental illness and addiction are ways many X-Men cope with no one getting who they are, with not being acknowledged, and with being made to feel wrong and judged.

Gary:

An implant creates a particular kind of vibration within us; it becomes something that impacts us and holds us. It has some sway over us in our life. The energetic implants related to ADD and ADHD are more potent and overwhelming than the examples given above, and for the most part, took place before this lifetime. The implants connected with ADD and ADHD keep kids in the frantic mode of this reality. They're not able to be calm, cool, and collected when they desire to be. So, they may be extremely active and always on the go physically, as if they're driven by a motor, or they may be so flooded with data and information they can't concentrate on much of anything, or both. They may also have a short fuse, as Anne said, and a tendency to erupt.

We've found that it's possible to remove or undo these implants using a process from Access Consciousness that can be done by Access Consciousness facilitators. I worked with an eight-year-old boy with ADD while he was watching TV. He felt me tap into him (without actually touching his body), and he turned around and said, "What are you doing?"

I said, "Just clearing some stuff that's making your life difficult."

He said, "Oh," and went back to watching TV. He could feel me every time I touched into him and ran another set of implants. In a few minutes, I ran all the implants off.

The next day, his mother called me, hysterical, "Put them back in place! He's been outside all day long, cutting a refrigerator box into a house. I liked it better when he hung on my shirt tails all the time, wanting my attention. He was my baby. You've taken away him being my baby."

"I said, 'Sorry, honey, I can't do that. I can't put them back in place.

Once they're gone, they're gone. You'd better get used to him the way he is."

Taking on Other People's Energy

These kids are psychically aware, so in addition to the implants, a lot of the so-called hyperactivity they exhibit has to do with taking on everybody else's energy as well as their own, and in a calm situation, they can be different. Kids with ADHD have a propensity to pick up the angst and worry of people around them. They are likely to have a parent or a stepparent who is a worrier, so they have a tendency to perceive this angst and worry dynamically.

Anne:

I recently did a session with a seven-year-old boy and his dad. The dad's wife, the boy's stepmom, had recently left them. Since then, the boy had been having outbursts at school and at home. In the session, he could not sit still. He was in constant motion, often sitting upside down in the chair with his head close to the ground and his feet in the air. His dad started to reprimand him, saying, "Petey, you need to sit up and listen."

I quickly said, "Actually, he's really listening and participating in our conversation, and it's fine with me if he's not sitting still."

Many people might think it's a sign of disrespect for someone not to sit still, focus, and pay attention. What I saw was that the topic of our conversation was difficult for the boy and his dad, and Petey was coping in the best way he knew how. They were talking about their relationship and what life had been like since the boy's stepmom had left; it was a conversation they had not been able to have before.

As they talked about the changes that had occurred in their family, Dad became more peaceful, and as he did, Petey also settled down. He was still wiggly, but he was much calmer. If I had focused on his behaviors, none of that could have been possible. Dad would have become increasingly upset at not being able to control his son, and Petey would have become even more hyper.

In my view, Dad's acknowledgment of the changes going on in their lives was a key factor in shifting them both into a completely different space. Acknowledgement is magic. It validates our awareness.

There are also a number of tools given throughout the book that can be lifesavers when kids are picking up other people's energy, worry, emotions, thoughts, and feelings. Among my go-to favorites are:

- Whose perception is this?
- Who does this belong to?
- Return to Sender.
- Who are you doing this for?

Physical Activity

In addition to encouraging parents to allow their kids to multi-task when they do their homework and to use Access Consciousness tools and processing, I also stress the importance of physical activity, whether it's in the classroom, during recess, or after school. It helps all kids release their energy and sit calmly in the classroom for longer periods of time, and it makes a huge difference for those with ADD and ADHD.

Dain:

Get their bodies moving even if it's just walking around the block a few times. I'll go jogging, or I'll go swimming, or I'll go do pushups, or I'll lie on one of those roller things and roll out my muscles—all of those—and when I get up, I feel so much better.

Anne:

The parents of a very bright six-year-old boy who is on the mild/moderate end of the autism spectrum and who has also been diagnosed with ADHD purchased a trampoline and set it up it in their backyard. They report that there is a huge difference in their son's behavior when he plays on the trampoline regularly. He has fewer "edges" when he has regular time on the trampoline.

The mother of a seven-year-old girl with ADD reports a similar easing of symptoms when the girl swims regularly. She loves being in the water! She is on a swim team and is one of their best swimmers. Before becoming involved in swimming, the girl had frequent tantrums, struggled immensely at school, couldn't pay attention, and was generally miserable. Since she has discovered swimming, she is better able to handle daily ups and downs, she gets her homework done with relative ease, and she has much more self-confidence. She told me, "My body likes to swim!"

Kids who have ADD or ADHD do much better when they are able to be outdoors, spend time with animals, and run around and play. It's expansive for them. Their bodies love it. They don't do well when they're cooped up in small spaces. They need to be given permission to be on the move!

Questions to Ask Yourself:

And here are some questions for you as a parent:

- Do you play with your child?
- Do you love watching your child do what he or she loves to do?
- Do you have fun with your child?
- If not, would you like to?
- What if you could play with him or her?
- What would it be like to step beyond the place of your child being a problem, and into the space of celebrating the difference he or she is and enjoying your time together?
- What would it take?

- And what if you don't need to know ahead of time how it's going to turn out?

If you've not been playing much with your child, what do you do? What if you just start from where you are right now? Be present! Be you! You might say to your child:

"I love to watch you swim!"

"Can I watch you do that again?"

"Can I play with you?"

~ 15 ~

AVERTING UPSETS

*If behavior is a form of communication, what are kids saying
when they act out, throw a tantrum, or sob uncontrollably?*
- Anne Maxwell

Anne:

Kids can become upset and have outbursts for many reasons, yet
when upsets occur, many parents and teachers try to calm the child,
divert her, make him "snap out of it," or employ some other sort of
tactic to end the upset rather than be with the upset and wonder
what's going on in the child's world.

As I said in chapter eleven, one of the underlying principles of my
practice is that behavior is a form of communication, so whenever I
hear of children having outbursts, the first questions I ask are:

- What is this child saying?
- What is he or she telling us?

These questions, asked with curiosity, openness, and no point of
view, provide so much information about what is being communicated with the tantrum or upset. When I ask questions like these, I
get a sense of what's going on in the child's universe. Asking these
questions moves me beyond the place of "right" and "wrong" and

into the space of possibilities. It moves me beyond a facile explanation like "He throws a fit whenever he doesn't get his way," and into the space of wondering what's going on that's causing this degree of outburst over such a seemingly insignificant incident.

Another underlying principle of my practice is that people do the best they can with the tools and the information they have available to them at the time. Other questions I ask myself in the face of a child's upset are:

- Is this the best this child can do right now?
- If so, what's going on in his or her world that's creating this behavior?
- What's right about this behavior I'm not getting?

What if the behavior that seems so wrong is telling you something you absolutely need to know about your child? What if it's communicating a need your child has that you're not getting? What if you listened to that communication in a way that allowed you to change some things that would make life better for everyone concerned?

X-Men kids function so differently, and the way we respond to them needs to be tailored to who they are and what they require in order to do well. In my experience, many of the cognitive and behavioral interventions that work with other kids don't work well with these children. So, we need to discover what *does* work.

All kids are unique, and they respond in different ways, but I've found that there are a number of triggers for upsets that many kids have in common. These include frustration about how slow everything is moving, being "bossed" or told what to do, not having a choice, not being acknowledged, not being listened to, and being judged or criticized. X-Men kids also have upsets and outbursts that express other people's (unexpressed) anger.

When these things are addressed with kids—and when parents and teachers begin to use a different approach, kids' behavior really changes. Even though it may not seem possible in the moment, it *is* possible to avert upsets or to defuse them more quickly once they've gotten started. When this is done over time, the outbursts typically don't last as long, they occur less frequently, and they are less intense.

Too Slow

We have spoken in earlier chapters about how children with ADD, ADHD, OCD, and autism function more quickly than others do. They don't have to go from A to B to C in order to understand something. Oftentimes they can go from A to Z instantly, and when they are made wrong for that or are told they must slow down, they can become angry.

I experienced this for myself the other day. I went to the bank and had just a few minutes to purchase a money order. The bank teller was chatty. She was going on and on about the errands she was going to run after she got off work that day, and as she was chatting, she actually stopped doing what was required to produce the money order. I thought my head was going to explode! Needless to say, I did not have an outburst, but it was excruciating for me to slow myself down to meet her where she was. And surprisingly, when I slowed myself down, she sped up.

If your child is super-fast and tends to get frustrated about how slow everything is, you can ask him or her, "You know how fast you are? Can this other person keep up with you?" The awareness that the other person isn't able to keep up may change everything.

You can also say, "I wonder if you can know how fast you are and how much slower this other person is."

Or you could try, "Can you be at a speed that she or he can hear?" The use of *be* and *hear* doesn't fit with our usual definitions of those words—because they're about the energy. Sometimes parents don't get this—but kids do! Try it and see how they respond.

Having No Choice

Most adults dislike being "bossed" or told what to do. It leaves them with a sense that they have no choice. They find it demeaning and disempowering, and sometimes it makes them really mad! They want to be treated with respect and courtesy. The same is true for kids.

A mother told me about how her high-spirited, extremely bright four-year-old daughter started to throw a fit when the mother announced where they would be going for dinner that evening.

"No, I don't want to go there!" she emphatically told her mom.

As the little girl started to become more agitated, the mom suddenly remembered *she* had told the girl that she could choose the restaurant they would be going to. She said, "Honey! I just remembered that I told you that *you* could choose the restaurant. After I said that, our friends called and invited us to go with them, and I completely forgot what I'd told you. I'm so sorry!"

The father of the other family saw immediately what was transpiring. He knew that the girl loved milk shakes, and he said, "They have really good milk shakes. If we were to go there, maybe you could have one." The little girl changed her mind in an instant. She stopped fussing, went along willingly, and everyone had a great time.

What did these adults do that was so effective? They recognized that they had inadvertently taken away the girl's choice, they acknowledged they had done so, and they offered a fresh, new choice, which she was happy to accept.

Not Being Acknowledged

Kids also become upset when they are not acknowledged. A mother came to talk with me about her six-year-old son. The boy was not present, but she brought her almost three-year-old daughter with her. At the end of the session, as we were standing in the doorway, the mother had something more she wanted to tell me. As she was speaking to me, her daughter kept interrupting her. The mother, appearing increasingly uncomfortable, ignored her daughter, who became more and more persistent. She started to whine and walk out of the room by herself. I asked the mother if I could speak with her daughter. She looked surprised and said, "Yes."

I knelt next to the girl and asked her if she had something she would like to add. She looked at her mom and said, "Mommy, I love Jamie (her brother). We play." Her mom smiled, relaxed, and said, "Thank you."

What did the little girl know about her brother that she was trying to communicate to her mother? Could it be that even though her mom and her brother were struggling, she didn't see anything "wrong" with her brother? Or was it an invitation to her mom to play with Jamie, to be less intense with him? Or was she inviting her mom to a different space?

It was clear that the little girl wished to contribute to her mother and brother, and even though the contribution may not have been clear cognitively, energetically it was a game changer. Her mom shifted into a different space and dropped her focus on her "problems" with her son. The mother smiled at her, and they left holding hands.

Gary:

Acknowledging kids is vital. My youngest daughter always talks to her one-year-old boy as though he is an adult. She says things like, "Will you please put that away?" or "Will you do this, please?" And he will do it. He gets the concept of what she is saying, and she also thinks at him in pictures, so he knows what's being asked of him.

What if we knew that all kids are communicating telepathically and we treated them as though they were infinite beings with infinite capacity to understand? Do you think that would make a difference in the way they respond to the world?

There's no reason for kids with ADD, ADHD, autism and OCD to have any problem if we're willing to be more aware and acknowledge them as the infinite beings they are. We create problems when we insist that they conform to our plans and designs or demand that they change and become someone they are not.

Judgment

Anne:

Sometimes kids' upsets can be less visible. At times children appear to pull inside themselves, make themselves invisible, or have tears without sobs. These are children whose upsets take the form of despair. The eleven-year-old son of friends of ours was sent off for a week to stay with his uncle and aunt in Vermont. He is a sparkling, creative, aware, and sensitive boy. But the visit wasn't going well. According to the uncle and the aunt, he was homesick and counting the days until he could go home. His mother had told her brother (the boy's uncle) that the boy would love to go shooting and hiking with him, yet the boy declined every offer his uncle made to do those things.

I asked my friend to tell me about her brother, and in a halting and reluctant way, she said that he tended to be extremely judgmental and to blame everyone else when things didn't go well. She said, "It is not possible to do well or be good enough in his eyes. His criticisms are scathing."

Someone might ask why the boy's mother would send her son into such a hostile environment. As we talked, I discovered that they are a close-knit family that places value on loyalty, so it was difficult for her to acknowledge what was actually true about her brother. She saw her negative view of him as a judgment, even a form of betrayal. In fact, in this case, it wasn't a judgment at all; it was simply an awareness that he is unkind.

What was this boy saying by counting the days, then the hours, until he could return home? What was he telling everyone when he declined his uncle's invitations? Was he being disrespectful? Was he a "mama's boy" as his uncle had stated? Did he need "toughening up"? Or did he wither under the unrelenting judgment of his uncle? Was he actually homesick—or was that the easiest way he found to manage the stress of being in an environment where there was a lack of kindness?

The boy is not my client, so I didn't have an opportunity to talk with him. However, if I did, I would ask him questions so he could have more awareness about his uncle and himself. I would ask, "What do you know about your uncle?" and I would not try to talk him out of his knowing. I would acknowledge it.

I would point out the difference between *perceiving* the meanness and the lack of kindness and *feeling* as if he deserved them. I would talk with him about judgment and criticism, and the difference between perceiving the judgment as something that the uncle was doing versus taking it on or "owning" it as any kind of truth about himself.

I'd also say, "Any time someone judges you, it's because *they* are being or doing the thing they are judging you for. So, when someone judges you as being not good enough, it just indicates that *the other person* feels not good enough. They are projecting their judgment about themselves onto you. It's crazy—because it has nothing to do with the way you are. They are throwing the judgments they have of themselves onto you."

When I'm working with children who seem withdrawn, sad, or emotionally shut down, I often find that they have bought into criticism or judgments that have been projected onto them. Kids are so aware and so ready to "own" other people's feelings and judgments that even subtle or unspoken judgments can have a big impact on them.

Kids know so much more about what's going around them than they are given credit for. When they are not acknowledged for what they know, they doubt themselves, act out, or cry a lot. And when they are acknowledged, they thrive.

Not Listening to What Kids Have to Say

I was talking with the mother of a twelve-year-old boy who has been diagnosed with ADHD and also has some autistic traits. She said he has a temper that flares out of control with seemingly little to no provocation. He was becoming increasingly disrespectful to her— refusing to help around the house, sneering at her when she asked him to do chores, cussing at her, and sometimes punching holes in the walls. The boy's dad, who she had divorced six years earlier, used to intimidate her in a similar way, by threatening to destroy property and having angry outbursts. After the divorce, she decided she would not allow herself to be treated like that ever again. Her son's disrespect reminded her of the darker days of her marriage, and she told me that she was unwilling to live like that again.

She said that after one particularly troubling moment, she took her son to stay with his dad, who had agreed ahead of time to support her in this manner. When the son returned home, things went well for a couple of weeks. He helped around the house and accepted no for an answer. Then one afternoon when she was in a hurry, she began to lose patience with him, and in that impatient state, she shut down to him.

He said, "Mom, you're not listening to me,"

She realized that she wasn't listening and said, "You're right. I wasn't listening, and I will now. What were you trying to tell me?" She then listened to what he had to say, and afterwards, he thanked her.

She realized how frequently she had shut herself off from him and refused to listen to him and how angry that had made him. This experience turned out to be a turning point in their relationship.

Tool: Who Am I Being Right Now?

This is a tool that's useful any time you or your kids become upset or emotional about something. You simply ask: Who am I being right now? Then ask: And, if I were being me, who would I be? You don't have to have an answer for who you are being. Just ask the question. You will have the awareness that you are not being you, and that's enough to shift into a different space.

It's a great tool to use with your kids when they are throwing a tantrum or doing trauma and drama. When you ask your child mid-tantrum, "Who are you being right now?" they might yell at you. But they will have the awareness that they are not being themselves, and this awareness will make it more difficult to continue the tantrum with the same gusto.

Whose Anger Is It?

In a class that Gary gave, the aunt of a twenty-one-year-old young man who has been diagnosed with autism described her nephew's struggles with a short temper. She told us he frequently flew off the handle and had recently lost a job because of his angry explosions. She said he is incredibly aware and intuitive, and described him as a healer. "He's got an amazing ability to heal," she said, "he's just unhappy."

Gary asked her whether the unhappiness was his, and she said, "No, the unhappiness is not his; it belongs to his parents."

Gary then asked whether he was trying to heal his parents' unhappiness.

"Yes," she responded, "he takes on his parents' unhappiness in an attempt to heal it."

Gary said, "You might ask him whether the explosion is his anger or whether it is the awareness he has of other people's anger and how they really want to explode but won't let themselves. Ask him whether he is capable of expressing what other people cannot."

In my practice, parents bring in their kids because of the kids' behavior. In clinical language, the person who is brought in for therapy is known as the "identified patient." Like this young man, many times, the kids are simply acting out what others in the family are unwilling to express. As Dain says, they are the ones who are capable of expressing what other family members repress and suppress.

Tool: Destroy and Uncreate Your Relationship

Unfortunately, upsets often persist long after they are "over." Kids tend to get stuck in decisions and conclusions they make that relate to the upset, and these can really derail a relationship.

This doesn't have to be the case if you destroy and uncreate your relationship with your child every day. You destroy and uncreate everything about who, what, where, when, why, and how you think the *child* is and everything about who, what, where, when, why, and how you are with the child, as well as everything about who, what, where, when, why, and how the *child* thinks *you* are with him or her.

Let's say you and your child have had some difficult moments, arguments, or conflicts during the day, and you would like to be in a different space with him or her. Or let's say you had a wonderful day and would like even more ease and joy to show up. In the evening before going to bed, say, "I destroy and uncreate everything my relationship was with my child today and in the past."

When you destroy and uncreate your relationship every night, you get to create your relationship anew every day, which means you're on the creative edge of a different possibility. You won't bring your upsets, decisions, and conclusions into the new day. You will be able to generate something fresh and new with your kids. If you do this every day, you will have a different kind of relationship with them. They will be able to talk to you about things they have never talked about before, and you will be able to talk with them about things you always wanted to and never did. This tool puts you in a constant state of generating or creating a relationship instead of functioning from old points of view. It is one of my favorite tools of Access Consciousness, and I use it daily.

Tool: Destroy and Uncreate All the Projections and Expectations You Have of Your Relationship

A variation of the "destroy and uncreate your relationship" tool is to destroy and uncreate all the projections and expectations you have of your relationship with your children, the kids in your classroom, your spouse, or anyone else. I like to do this every morning.

When you destroy and uncreate your relationship with someone—as well as the expectations and projections you have of that person, you destroy and uncreate the limitations of the past and the solidity of the future you are creating. You are able to be in the present with such ease, and from that space, you create a different future.

Trina and Aaron

My friend, Trina, the occupational therapist who works in the public school system, told me a story about Aaron, a fifteen-year-old boy who has autism. He is non-verbal and communicates on an iPad. He requires assistance to type; someone has to put their hand on top of his to steady it in order for him to type, and it can be a slow process. His mind works at the speed of light, and this process can be enormously frustrating to him.

Trina sees Aaron daily. She told me that two or three times a day, he would drop to the floor and throw a tantrum. Often he would pull the teacher's and paraprofessional's hair.

One day when he was calm, she asked him, "What do you know about the times when you throw tantrums?" He typed in "math and social studies." Trina said that both classes were held in the same classroom with the same teacher.

She asked him what else he knew. He replied, "My teacher thinks I'm stupid." She asked if the teacher had told him that verbally, and he typed, "No, but that's what she thinks. I can hear it in my head."

Trina asked him whether he thought he was stupid and he replied, "No, but my teacher does."

Then she inquired, "Do you know how amazingly brilliant you are in the way you perceive and see things? It's so different from the way others perceive and see things."

He replied, "Yes, but she doesn't understand."

She asked whether he could destroy and uncreate his relationship with that teacher. She said, "People can project their judgments onto us, and maybe those are her judgments of herself for not knowing how to communicate with you. If you destroy and uncreate your relationship with her every day, you will be destroying and uncreating all of the judgments she has put on you each day. Are you able to do that?"

He replied, "Yes."

She asked him, "Do you understand?" to which he responded, "YES TRI-NA!"

That it was the first time he had ever written her name. She said she had been amazed at the amount of information he had given to her, since they had communicated on the iPad and it had required so much time, effort, and persistence—as well as vulnerability. Immediately after that, Aaron's hair pulling and floor-flopping behaviors decreased from two or three times a day to once or twice a week.

ALLOWANCE

Your point of view creates your reality.
Reality does not create your point of view.
- Dr. Dain Heer

Gary:

When you are in a place where you can be in allowance of people as they are, it's rare and precious to them. They want you to stay with them; they don't want you to leave. They like having you around because you don't look at them with judgment—and when you look at someone without judgment, you are the most seductive thing that ever walked the Earth. All kinds of things become possible. Your ability to be in allowance is a tremendous gift.

Anne:

Allowance is stepping out of the space of thinking there are right and wrong ways to be and do things. You simply perceive things as they are. When you step into a space of allowance, everything becomes more clear and you have the freedom to make other choices.

Gary:

You can align and agree with a point of view, or you can resist and react to a point of view. That's the polarity of this reality. Or you can be in allowance. If you are in allowance, you are the rock in the middle of the stream. Thoughts, beliefs, attitudes, and considerations come at you and they go around you because to you, they're just an interesting point of view. If, on the other hand, you go into alignment and agreement or resistance and reaction to that point of view, you get caught up in the stream of insanity and you go along for a ride. That's not the stream you want to be in. You want to be in allowance. Total allowance is: Everything is just an interesting point of view.

Alignment and Agreement

Anne:

When I first heard Gary talk about allowance, it changed everything for me. I saw how I had spent so much of my life trying to fit in. I had tried to align and agree with what everyone else thought, all to no avail. I was continuously getting washed away in the stream of other people's viewpoints.

When I was in third grade, a man who lived in our town was running for the U.S. Senate. Our teacher told the class that because this guy was from our town, that our parents should vote for him. I immediately went into agreement with her point of view. "Oh, yeah, that's right. Our parents *should* vote for him."

When I repeated that viewpoint to my mom, she said, "Just because he lives next door to us, doesn't mean we're going to vote for him. I would *never* vote for that man."

I then went into agreement with *that* point of view, "Right! We don't have to vote for him just because he lives by us!" and when I repeated it to my teacher (with all the sarcasm and scorn my mother had expressed), she made me stay in the classroom during recess and copy pages out of the dictionary—because I had been disrespectful.

It's very easy for parents of X-Men kids to fall into the trap of aligning and agreeing with all the "experts" about their kids' "disabilities" and the "right" way to parent them and/or educate them. It makes a world of difference when you shift out of alignment and agreement: "Oh, yes, that must be right," and instead move into allowance: "Hmm, that's an interesting point of view. What's true for me and my child?"

Resistance and Reaction

When Gary first talked about allowance, I also saw how people spent their lives resisting and reacting to what everyone else thought, said, and did. I recognized that I had done my share of this as well. As a kid, any time someone told me I couldn't do or have something, I did everything within my power to do or have it. Once when I was seven years old, my mom pointed out a full-page newspaper advertisement of children's shoes. She told me I could have any of them I liked—except one particular pair. I threw a fit, cried, and carried on about how that was the only pair I would consider wearing. After a while, she "gave in" and purchased a pair of those shoes for me. I learned years later that the "forbidden" shoes were the ones she wanted me to wear. She had manipulated me, knowing I would resist and react! To this day, I'm sometimes still like that. Someone tells me, "No," and my initial response is "Watch me!"

However, thanks to Gary, I saw that there was another choice. It was being in allowance—perceiving everything as an interesting point of view—and this has made a huge difference for me in my relationships and in my work.

Being in Allowance as a Parent

What if you did not demand that your kids align and agree with your points of view? What if you could give them permission to have their own points of view and to change their viewpoints as they see fit? What if you could give your kids permission to be who they are?

Being in allowance with all kids is essential—and it's imperative in dealing with X-Men kids. Kids on the autism spectrum, for example, can have odd behaviors. Rather than having a strong point of view about whether they are right or wrong, if you can ask questions and tap into what they are saying, seemingly intractable situations and difficulties can shift.

Being in a space of allowance does not mean you become a doormat and allow your kids to run you over. It does not mean that you say *yes* to every demand they make of you. And it does not mean that you exclude yourself from the equation.

Being in allowance definitely doesn't mean that you don't say *no*. Sometimes *no* is exactly what's called for. And if your child explodes, what if you could allow the explosion to occur and not feel responsible for it? It can take practice not to feel humiliated in the grocery store when your child has a tantrum and flops around on the floor. However, when you are in the space of total allowance of your child and what he is choosing in the moment—when you see his choice as an interesting point of view—there is no one to push back against, and typically the outbursts don't last as long.

"Okay" is a perfectly appropriate energetic response to a tantrum (not "Oohhh-kaay!"), just "Okay" with the energy of "if this is what you are choosing, okay."

Dain:

If you have no judgment in your point of view, you will have no limitation in how your reality can show up, because judgment is the great limiter.

Gary:

Any time you take a fixed point of view about anything, you are creating an anchor that keeps you stuck where you are.

Anne:

When you don't have a point of view about the choices your kids make, it frees you up to ask questions and step beyond any pre-conceived notions you and others might have about what they are choosing.

Dain:

The point of view you take is always your choice. Changing it to something different because it works better for you is also your choice. You don't ever have to be stuck with the point of view you currently have—about anything.

Anne:

Nor do your kids. When you go into allowance, you energetically allow kids to change their points of view.

Recently I facilitated a class that was attended by a mom and her twenty-one-month-old son. At one point, he picked up a very large, heavy water bottle they had brought with them, and tottering under its weight, he hoisted it up over his head to get a drink. There was just a tiny bit of water left in it, and instead of going into his mouth, most of the water went down the front of his shirt and onto the floor.

He put the bottle down and said, "Mama…Moh!"

His mom looked at him and said, "Look, you've spilled it all over your shirt and onto the floor. No, you can't have any more water in the bottle."

At that point, he did what he always does when his mom says no or tries to control him. He looked her in the eyes and screamed.

I asked his mom, "Whose shirt is it, anyway?"

She smiled, relaxed, dropped her point of view, and said to him, "Okay, you can have more water in the bottle."

Since Mom was involved with another class participant in a project, I offered to get more water for him. The water was very cold. I put about three fingers of it in the bottle and handed it back to him. There were ice cubes in it and he could see them. He ran back to his mom, put the bottle on the floor, rubbed the front of his shirt: "Nooo, Mama…Nooo, Mama!" He knew he didn't want any of that cold water on his chest.

He did not attempt to drink water out of the bottle then or for the rest of the weekend. Instead he asked me to go with him to the table where the water was and pour some into a small plastic cup for him.

As long as his Mom had the point of view that he shouldn't drink out of the water bottle, his only choice was to push back and scream. The minute she dropped her point of view about all of that, he got to tap into what he would create by drinking the ice cold water out of the huge bottle—ice water down the front of his shirt—and he choose something else.

~ 17 ~

CHOICE

There should always be choice for kids.
You need to recognize that they're choosing what they are choosing
to get a result that they think will change something.
~ Gary Douglas

Anne:

There is a widespread belief that kids with so-called disabilities aren't able to make "good" choices, and adults aren't often willing to let them make choices about the day-to-day things in their lives. It may seem to many kids and the adults who interact with them that the kids don't have choice about anything—but what if they actually do?

Kids actually make choices continuously. They choose whether to be grumpy (or not), whether to be silly (or not), whether to bang their head on the floor (or not), whether to step into a different space (or not), whether to go along with a request we make (or not).

When we are in the space of allowance of their choices, they get to tap into the energy of what they are creating and they can continue to choose what they've chosen—or to make a different choice.

A friend who works with X-Men kids in the public school system points out that choice exists even in the midst of upsets and outbursts. She told me about one of her middle-school-age students with autism. He was nonverbal but communicated energetically all the time—except nobody ever listened. This young man had frequent angry outbursts.

She said that many times when she arrived in the classroom to work with him, he would have already bolted from the class or had a physically aggressive outburst. One day just before she arrived, he had attempted to flee and had almost put his hand through a window. When she walked into the room, he was being restrained on a mat by two para-professionals to ensure his safety.

She looked at the student and said, "Hey, you're creating being more controlled. Is that really what you'd like to create?"

He looked her in the eye—and this was someone who didn't make eye contact. He said, "Hmmah," stopped resisting, and became calm instantly. He was up and back to work in seconds.

He made a choice.

How Do You Choose?

When we speak about choice, we're not talking about some sort of cognitive process where you think long and hard about something, carefully weigh the pros and cons, and then choose. We are not talking about right answer and wrong answer or good choice and bad choice. The "choice" we're talking about has to do with energy, not cognition.

So, how do you choose? You just choose!

As an adult, you choose to get up when the alarm goes off (or not). You choose to make an obscene gesture at the driver who cut you off (or not). You choose to go along with your boss's request that you stay late to finish a project (or not). You choose how to respond to every situation in your life. You just choose. It's the same for your kids.

As Gary says, "Everything is just a choice."

And your choice doesn't need to last forever. If you don't like the choice you made, you can choose something else. What if you could let your kids—and yourself—choose, and then choose again?

Choice Creates Awareness

When you choose, you become aware of what your choice is creating now and what it will create in the future, just like the little boy in the previous chapter who tapped into what he would create by attempting to drink ice-cold water out of the huge water bottle. He had the awareness of what each choice would create, and he chose the one that worked best for him.

We facilitate this awareness for kids when we are in allowance of what they choose. And we invite them to a different possibility when we ask them questions.

A ten-year-old-boy I will call David, was brought to see me because he had frequent explosive outbursts. I was told by his mother that he was quick to explode, become defensive, hurl insults, groan, and hit his head with his fists in frustration. He was a brilliant kid, and he got impatient when people either couldn't or didn't keep up with him or when they didn't acknowledge him.

Because David had been punished, reprimanded, and faulted for his outbursts so often, his view of himself was that there was something wrong with him. And because his life didn't seem to change much, he seemed resigned to being wrong, not having friends, and being in trouble constantly. He was hopeless that things could ever get better and told me he saw no way out. His mother was also in despair and would project into the future and warn him how difficult and unhappy his life would become if he didn't get a grip on himself now. Neither one of them believed that David had choices.

When David and I talked, he portrayed himself as a victim of mean, unpleasant kids, parents who didn't understand him, and teachers who were out to get him. I asked him lots of questions about his life at home and at school, and we talked about the notion that he actually had choice. Even though he resisted initially, he was able to acknowledge that maybe he did have choice.

Over time, David began to make different choices. He became less at the effect of kids, teachers, and his parents. He was less reactive to what others did or said and less prone to outbursts. And when he did have them, they did not last as long and were less intense. For example, if the boy who lived next door, one of his few playmates, was not able to play, instead of becoming upset, David was able to take it in stride and move on.

What did I do to facilitate this change? I asked him questions. I did not demand "answers," I acknowledged whatever he told me, and I had no point of view about the choices he made.

A boy in David's class was his nemesis. This boy provoked him constantly, and David bought into it most of the time. One day, the boy talked a mutual friend of theirs out of inviting David to his birthday party. In my office, David plotted revenge.

Unlike almost everyone in his life, I had no point of view about what he was going to choose to do. When he would plot revenge in other instances, people would jump in and try to talk him out of his plans, which would only escalate him. Instead, I simply acknowledged everything he was saying and then said, "Could I ask you a question?"

"Yes."

"If you carry out these plans, what will your life be like in a day? In a week? In a month? And if you don't carry out these plans and instead do something different, what would your life be like in a day? In a week? In a month?"

Even though he initially claimed his life would be so much better if he were able to have revenge, he tapped into the energy of what he would create by making each choice he contemplated, and as it turned out, he chose a more measured response.

David told me later that the boy was irritated that David did not erupt as was his pattern, and as a result, did not get in trouble.

"So, who got the last word, anyway?" I asked him.

He grinned.

Being in allowance of kids' choices is essential, but unfortunately many parents and teachers engage in right and wrong thinking or have strong points of view about children. When this occurs, kids often miss out on the chance to make choices and be aware of what their choice has created.

One summer, I worked briefly with a mom and her five-year-old and two-and-a-half-year-old sons. She was concerned about the older boy. She told me that he played roughly with his younger brother, so she brought both boys to the session so I could witness this. As she described the older boy to me, it seemed that she was looking for me to validate all the decisions and conclusions she had reached about him. It was important for her to have answers and to be in control. She was anything but in allowance of her two boys.

I observed as the brothers played easily and kindly with each other; occasionally the older boy gave toys to his younger brother. At one point, when his little brother tried to take a truck away from him, the older boy let him have it. He was so different from the way his mother had described him!

She said nothing when this occurred. It was as if she wasn't able to see beyond her decisions and conclusions.

There was a step stool in the room, which the two-and-a-half year old dragged over to the window. Mom started to stand up in alarm, worried that he might fall. I smiled at Mom and quietly asked her to stay where she was. I had no point of view about the little boy being on the step stool, as I was close to him and I knew I would be able to catch him if he started to fall. He turned around and looked at me. I smiled at him and remained still, energetically giving him permission to explore. Very carefully, he crawled up onto the stool and stood up. He turned around again with a broad smile on his face, and I applauded him. He then reversed his motions, and slowly stepped back down onto the rug.

From my point of view, he was demonstrating that choice creates awareness. He chose to climb up onto the stool, and in choosing, he knew that he could stand on the stool without falling. When he was given the space to choose for himself, he did—with full awareness of what that would create.

Mom could have applauded him as well—but instead she was furious. She said, "He could have fallen! He's clumsy and he falls a lot. I can't believe you let him be so unsafe."

She did not bring the boys back to see me again. That was her choice.

~ 18 ~

THE CLEARING STATEMENT

You are the only one who can unlock the points of view that have you trapped. What we are offering here with the clearing process is a tool you can use to change the energy of the points of view that have you locked into unchanging situations.

~ Gary Douglas

Gary:

Throughout this book, and especially in the next section about your role as a parent, we ask a lot of questions, and some of those questions might twist your head around a little bit. That's our intention. The questions we ask are designed to get your mind out of the picture so you can get to the energy of a situation.

Once the question has twisted your head around and brought up the energy of a situation, we'll ask if you are willing to destroy and uncreate that energy—because stuck energy is the source of barriers and limitations. Destroying and uncreating that energy will open the door to new possibilities for you.

This is your opportunity to say, "Yes, I'm willing to let go of whatever is holding that limitation in place."

That will be followed by some weird-speak we call the clearing statement:

Everything that is times a godzillion, will you destroy and un-create it all? Right and Wrong, Good and Bad, POD and POC, All 9, Shorts, Boys, and Beyonds®.

You don't have to understand the words of the clearing statement for it to work because, as we've said, it's about the energy. You don't even have to use the words in the clearing statement to release the energy of your limitations. Once the question is asked, you can simply say, "And everything I read in that book about X-Men," and this will clear the energy, if that is your intention. However, if you'd like to know more about what the words in the clearing statement mean, they are defined at the end of this book.

Basically, with the clearing statement, we're going back to the energy of the limitations and barriers that have been created. We're looking at the energies that keep us from moving forward and expanding into all of the spaces that we would like to go. The clearing statement is simply a short speech that addresses the energies that are creating the limitations and contractions in our life.

Anne:

When I first heard the clearing statement, it struck me that it made *no sense!* Yet even though it sounded silly, it worked. And it worked instantly. As Gary says, it isn't necessary to understand the words with your logical brain. The words are designed to bypass your logical mind. I remember the first time I heard Gary say, "Since the first language is energy, even if we were to say the clearing statement in a language you do not speak, it would still work." That's the magic of it.

What does clearing mean? It's getting rid of stuff. It's letting go. Most of the limitations and places we are stuck have been created by our insanity—by doing the same thing over and over again and expecting a different result.

The clearing process can be done in different ways, but it usually starts with a question—and sometimes it's a head-twisting question like "What's the value of holding on to everything I want to get rid of?" As you ask the question, the energy of the insanity of holding onto everything you want to get rid of comes up.

You acknowledge and receive the energy that comes up, and you express your willingness to destroy and uncreate it. By so doing, you are destroying and uncreating all the ways and places you bought the limitations as real and true.

The final step is to repeat the clearing statement.

> *Right and Wrong, Good and Bad, POD and POC, All 9, Shorts, Boys, and Beyonds.*

So, here it is:

> *What's the value of holding onto everything I want to get rid of? Everything that is, I destroy and uncreate it all. Right and Wrong, Good and Bad, POD and POC, All 9, Shorts, Boys, and Beyonds.*

Gary:

The more you run the clearing statement, the deeper it goes and the more layers and levels it can unlock for you. If a lot of energy comes up for you in response to a question, you may wish to repeat the process numerous times until the subject being addressed is no longer an issue for you.

You can choose to do this or not; we don't have a point of view about that, but we do want to invite you to try it and see what happens.

19

WHAT IS YOUR ROLE AS A PARENT?

What if you, as a parent, are perfect just the way you are?
~ Dr. Dain Heer

Gary:

Parents often misidentify and misapply their role as parents to include things like having to know it all, having to provide kids with a list of rules and regulations, and having to control their behavior. Many parents believe other people will judge them based on what their kids do.

Anne:

And what if many people *do* judge you based on what your kids do? What if many people are incredibly judgmental and will judge you no matter what you say or do? And what if you didn't override your knowing in favor of someone else's opinion or judgment?

Gary:

Are you attempting to live the American (or the Australian or the Italian or whatever it is) Dream, where you are a really cool person who marries the perfect wife or husband, lives in the perfect house with a white picket fence, and raises the perfect kids who everybody loves and admires you for having?

Would you give up being a cool person—and start to be an aware person instead? Everything you have done to make yourself cool instead of aware, will you destroy and uncreate it all? Right and Wrong, Good and Bad, POD and POC, All 9, Shorts, Boys, and Beyonds.

How much judgment do you have to do to determine whether you have a perfect life? A lot or a little? Megatons!

Everything you have done to judge whether or not you are creating the perfect life you decided you were supposed to create, whether it is based on you and your relationship, your kids, the money you have or the money you don't have, or anything else, and anything you are doing to judge you for not creating the perfect life, will you destroy and uncreate it please? Right and Wrong, Good and Bad, POD and POC, All 9, Shorts, Boys, and Beyonds.

Dain:

Have you ever noticed that when you are doing judgment, you never come out on the winning side? Have you ever observed that you never judge you for being much greater than you are?

Gary:

Or better than you are? Or more wonderful than you are?

Dain:

You always judge yourself as less-than. You judge you as more messed up than you are, you judge you as having more problems and all that sort of thing.

Gary:

Do you blame yourself for what you have decided is your kid's disability—or what has been labeled a disability?

Everywhere you have done blame, shame, regret, or guilt for your kid's having this ability instead of a disability, will you now destroy and uncreate it all? Right and Wrong, Good and Bad, POD and POC, All 9, Shorts, Boys, and Beyonds.

Would you give up being a problem as a reality? Thank you. Right and Wrong, Good and Bad, POD and POC, All 9, Shorts, Boys, and Beyonds.

And would you be willing to see that your kids are not a problem, but a possibility—especially if you have kids who have ADD, ADHD, autism, or OCD? Everything that is, will you destroy and uncreate it all? Right and Wrong, Good and Bad, POD and POC, All 9, Shorts, Boys, and Beyonds.

How Were You Treated as a Kid?

Gary:

Most of us haven't had role models for parenting that were nurturing and caring, and as a result, we tend to treat our kids, ourselves, and all the other people in our life the way we *were* treated—not the way we *should have been* treated. Dain provided a great example of this after he got a huge, new TV with surround-sound stereo that knocks you out of your chair.

Dain:

Gary's daughter, Grace, said, "Dain, can my friend and I watch a DVD on your system?"

I had a weird reaction. I thought, "What do you mean? It's *my* system."

Why wouldn't I let her use it? Why not? I could have said, "Yes, please enjoy it. Have a good time." Did I do that? No. I got weird and mistrustful. I said, "Yes, but just this once."

Gary:

Right after Dain said that, he turned to me and said, "Geez, I don't feel good about what I just said. What do I need to look at differently?"

I asked, "Were you a bad kid?"

He said, "No."

I asked, "Did you take care of your parents' stuff?"

He said, "All the time."

I asked, "Did you break things and have wild-ass parties?"

Dain said, "Nope. Never. I took care of everything all the time." (That's because he was the only adult in his family, but that's a different story.)

I said, "What if you treated Grace the way you should have been treated instead of the way you were treated?"

Dain:

I said, "Whoa." I had to look at that. My dad got remarried when I was six and my stepmother distrusted me from the moment she met me, even though I was one of those kids who would take care of everything for everyone. After my dad got married, I lived in the fairy tale I've always wanted to live in, with a wicked stepmother.

Gary:

Dain used to get up in the morning to fix his mother's coffee for her, and he'd serve it to her in bed.

Dain:

And sometimes breakfast too. My mom trusted me, but my stepmother was so distrustful that she didn't want me to stay in the house alone. I'm not sure what she thought, but she wouldn't trust me with the stuff in the house and she wouldn't trust me with the cars. I was a good kid, but that's not the way I was treated. Once Gary and I started to talk about it, I noticed I treated other people in my life that same way—with distrust.

Gary:

I asked Dain whether he treated himself that way as well. He said *yes,* he did. Most of us do this. We treat ourselves the way we were treated. We figure that has to be the right way because that's what our parents did. How are you treating yourself in your life? Are you treating yourself the way you should have been treated—or the way you were treated?

Dain:

And are you treating your kids the way you should have been treated based on your awareness and how cool you were—or are you treating them the way you were treated, simply because you were treated that way?

> *Everything that is, will you destroy and uncreate it all? Right and Wrong, Good and Bad, POD and POC, All 9, Shorts, Boys, and Beyonds.*

"I'm Never Going to Be Like My Mother"
Gary:

We tend to think that the other side of treating our kids they way we were treated is to declare, "I'm never going to be like my parents and do the things they did!" I did this. When I was very young, I decided that I was never going to treat my kids the way my mother treated me.

Once, when my oldest son was a teenager, I was awakened at 3:00 in the morning by the sound of loud talking and laughing in the living room. It was my son and his friends. I knew he had to be to work at six in the morning, so what did I do? I got up, stomped out into the living room, and righteously said, "Young man, you are not being responsible..."

No sooner were the words out of my mouth than I realized I was being just like my mother. I also realized that my son wasn't going to pay any more attention to me than I paid to my mother. I stopped in the middle of my sentence and said, "...and my mother said this to me and I didn't pay attention to her, either. Goodnight," and I went back to bed.

It doesn't work to decide you're not going to be like your parents. If you decide that you don't want to be like them, you'll just have to duplicate them—like I did. What does work, however, is being aware.

What if the greatest gift you can give to your kids is the gift of awareness?

Being Careful vs. Being Aware

A lot of parents are focused on wanting to keep their kids safe. They see this as their job, and I agree it's an important part of their role. The question is "What's the best way to keep them safe?" Is it to feverishly look out for them and warn them to be careful? Or is it to teach them that they can take care of themselves by being aware?

When my youngest son was about eighteen months old, we were at a park, and he decided he wanted to go on a very tall slide with the big kids. He started climbing the ladder. I was about twenty feet away, thinking at him, "Be careful, Sky, be careful." He got about three-quarters of the way up the ladder and called out, "Dad, I *am* being careful."

He was picking up my thoughts. I realized you have to be aware of what you're thinking at kids—because they pick it up. Don't tell them to be careful. Tell them to be aware. Awareness encompasses everything around them. When they're aware, they don't have to be careful, because they will know what to do.

Parents tell their kids things like "Be careful. Don't talk to strangers." I learned not to do that. I said, "Be aware. If something doesn't feel right, get the hell out of there—no matter who it is. Even if it's somebody you know, don't do anything with anybody that doesn't feel right to you, even if you know them."

Dain:

There is such a big difference between *aware* and *careful*. Has anybody ever told you to be careful? What does that mean? Be paranoid? That's the only option you have. *Careful* means paranoid. It means full of care or anxious. Being careful paralyzes you.

Aware is "Hey, everything is cool, everything is cool, everything is cool. Uh-oh. Wait a minute. What's that? That doesn't feel so good. I'm going to pay more attention to it or get away from it." Being aware gives you more options and lets you take action or get the hell out of there.

Gary:

When you tell somebody to be careful, they have to assume they are missing something that might harm them. In our work with horses, we've discovered that if you are fearful around them, they automatically assume they have missed something. They become nervous and paranoid. They figure they should have been able to see whatever is going on that made you fearful. The same thing applies with your kids. When you say, "Be careful," they assume there is something they have missed, and will always miss, and that they have no other choice but to miss it.

After my ex-wife and I divorced, she went to Mexico with my youngest daughter. Now, my ex-wife is somewhat volatile…

Dain:

Just a bit. She's kind of like a tornado, a hurricane, and an atom bomb put together with a candy-coated shell. I'll be quiet now; carry on.

Gary:

So, my daughter went to Mexico with her mother. She was about sixteen. One day when I was talking with her on the phone, she mentioned that her mother was constantly telling her to be careful. She found it annoying and asked me about it.

I said, "Honey, you don't need to be careful; you just need to be aware. You speak beautiful Spanish, but you don't understand every word that's being said. If you're aware, you'll definitely get the energy of any situation and you'll know when it's time to leave. If somebody wants to fool you, they'll use words you don't understand. So, don't be careful; be in your awareness."

Don't take care; be aware. A lady told me a story about her son. She kept telling him to be aware. One day he was standing near a building in a city, and he thought, "I don't want to be standing here. I want to be standing over there." He moved—and then something fell off the building and crushed the sidewalk where he had been standing. If he'd been being careful, he would have been looking around for who was going to "get" him; he wouldn't have been aware that he needed to move because something was coming down from above.

> So, everything you've bought yourself and everything you've locked into your body about being careful or through being careful, will you destroy and uncreate it and return it all to sender? Right and Wrong, Good and Bad, POD and POC, All 9, Shorts, Boys, and Beyonds.

"Did You Break the Cement?"

The other thing is when your kids fall down, don't assume they've hurt themselves, then run over to them and ask if they're all right. Pain is a creation, not a reality. When my kids would fall down on the cement, I'd walk over and ask, "Did you break the cement?" They'd look up at me, say *no*, and run off to play. No bruises, no scabs, no bumps.

If I had gone over and said, "Oh no! Are you all right, honey?" they would have cried and gotten a big bump on their head.

If you ask, "Are you hurt?" they'll always be hurt. If you ask, "Did you break the cement?" they'll say *nope* and happily run off.

Parenting with Awareness

Parenting with awareness is the willingness to recognize that you don't have all the answers and that you must learn to ask the question that will wake up your child. Awareness is recognizing that you cannot control your child; all you can do is manipulate him or her. You can manipulate your kids into doing the things you would like them to do and not doing the things you would not like them to do. Awareness is also the willingness to see what works for them.

Parents sometimes ask me about disciplining kids. I reply that I was raised with an occasional whack, so naturally, I tried that with my kids. It didn't work. I began to realize that the only effective discipline is to let kids know what is going to happen when they do something. Then let them choose what they want to do. Giving them a choice is always the best option. I would give my kids a choice of three or four things that they could choose, three of which were not nice. I'd say, "You can have this, this, this, or this. And if you don't choose this one, you're going to be unhappy."

Dain:

When Gary's kids were young, he wouldn't say, "Don't touch the stove." Instead he'd say, "If you touch that hot stove, it's going to hurt a lot." The kids would get close enough to feel the heat and they'd say, "Oh, maybe Dad's right." He didn't tell them not to touch it; he simply let them know what was going to happen if they did.

Gary:

When my youngest son was nine months old, we'd go to the grocery store and he would stand up in the shopping cart. He would not sit down in the little seat. One day as we were walking around the store, I said, "You know what, young man? You really ought to sit down because if you fall out on this hard floor, you're going to crack your head and that's not going to feel good." And he looked at me, went "Oh!" and sat down.

An older lady who was standing nearby started to laugh. She said, "That's the weirdest thing I've ever seen. I've never heard anybody talk to a baby like that."

I said, "He's got a small body, but he's an infinite being."

It's amazing what a difference it makes to explain things to children, even when they're very young. They will listen.

No More Than Four Rules

When you get to the point where they are teenagers, never give them more than four rules. With my youngest daughter, the rules were 1) No drinking and driving—because I know you're going to drink; 2) You can drink at home and your friends can drink at home as long as none of you leave and go anywhere else; 3) No boys can spend the night when I'm not home; and 4) Never more than three boys in the house at one time. The one thing I know about boys is that when they get together, they can get really rowdy and crazy at the wrong time.

I also asked, "Would you please call me and tell me when you're coming home—because I don't go to sleep until I know that you are here. Would you please do this for me? It would be really helpful." That wasn't a rule; it was a request. Those were the only things I asked of her. Then I said, "If you don't show up, I'm going to be out looking for you."

Dain:

One night Grace called Gary and said, "Dad, call me and tell me I have to come home."

He said, "Okay," and he called right back and said, "Grace, you've got to come home," and she came home.

Gary asked her, "What was the deal?"

She said, "We were at my friend's house and her parents were gone. There were three girls and two drunk boys and five more drunk boys coming over. That did not feel safe to me, and I wanted you to get me out of there."

Gary:

That's being aware rather than careful.

If you only have a few rules, kids will start to use their awareness, they will start to be present in their life, and they won't create the hideous situations that a lot of parents have to deal with. Trust your kid. If you trust your kids and you're willing to tell them that you trust them, it will create an amazing difference in the way they act.

Dain:

Are you who you are as a result of the restrictions your parents put on you—or the trust they put in you? I'd say that you are who you are pretty much because of the trust they put in you.

Gary:

Or did you just turn out well because you were cool in the first place?

Dain:

I used to think that I was so good in school and such a cool kid because of all the rules and restrictions my dad and stepmother imposed on me. I thought those were necessary to raise a kid. Later when I looked at it, I realized that the rules and restrictions had nothing to do with the way I turned out. I behaved the way I did because of me, despite the rules and restrictions.

Gary:

> *So, everything you've done not to recognize that none of the discipline imposed on you had to do with you, you were just cool to start with, and everything you've not been willing to know, be, perceive, and receive about that, will you now destroy and uncreate it all? Right and Wrong, Good and Bad, POD, POC, All 9, Shorts, Boys and Beyonds.*

Trying to Control Kids

I have four children. By the time my fourth child came along, I was so frigging tired that I couldn't consider the possibility of trying to control what she ate. I just said, "Eat anything you want, honey." She is now in her twenties and she eats the best of all my kids. How did that happen? I didn't try to control her. With my other kids, I made sure that everything was organic and that they didn't eat too much sugar. It was control, control, and control.

My youngest son had a friend named Matt who used to come to our house. We always had a tea service out, with a sugar bowl and things for preparing and serving tea when someone came over.

Every time Matt came over, I would find a big, messy pile of sugar outside the sugar bowl and all over the tray, and the sugar spoon would be crunchy with sugar. I knew Matt's parents forbade him to eat sugar, so I couldn't quite figure out how this mess happened. One day when he came over, I hid in the other room and waited to see what was going on.

I watched as he dug the sugar spoon into the sugar bowl and shoveled a spoonful of sugar into his mouth, then another and another. I stepped out and asked him, "Matt, what are you doing? Eating sugar out of my sugar bowl is not cool with me."

Matt looked at me like he was really scared.

I said, "You're not allowed to eat sugar at home, are you?"

He said, "No."

I asked, "What would happen if I told your dad?"

Matt said, "He would whip me."

I said, "I'm not going to tell your dad, but you have to make an agreement with me. I'll let you eat any kind of sugar you choose when you're at my house as long as you don't eat out of my sugar bowl."

He asked, "I can have anything?"

I said, "Yeah."

The next three times he came to our house, he loaded up on sugar like crazy, and after that, he forgot about it, because it was no longer forbidden to him. Suddenly the necessity of having it went away. We make a big mistake as parents when we forbid our kids to have things or to do things.

I made this mistake with my oldest daughter, who was supposedly allergic to dairy products and chocolate. We made sure that she only drank goat's milk and had no chocolate. We tried like heck to control what she ate. Then one day after she went away to summer camp, we decided to clean her room. Under the bed, in the closet, in every drawer and every other place you could think of, there were pieces of chocolate and crumbled up chocolate wrappers. She was sneaking the stuff all the time.

Be aware that if you forbid your children to do something, they are going to do it.

Dain:

Recognize that your kids are just like you. They are just as obnoxious as you are. What do you do when someone forbids you to do something—even if you are the one doing the forbidding? Have you ever tried to go on a fast? You tell yourself you can't eat. Then what do you want to do? Break the fast as soon as possible! All you can think of is eating.

Well, your kids are just like you. If you don't expect that your kids are going to be so different from you, you can ask, "Well, what would I have done in their shoes? What would I have done at their age?" You might get a clearer perspective on where they're functioning from. We tend to expect our kids to be the perfection we never were.

What if your children didn't have to be perfect?

Gary:

Or what if they are perfect just the way they are?

Dain:

What if they are perfect just the way they are, even if they have ADD, ADHD, OCD, autism or something else going on?

And what if you, as a parent, are perfect just the way you are? Do you believe that you have to be the perfect parent, the right parent, the good parent, and that if you are not the good parent, if you are not the perfect parent, your kids will die and go to hell or they'll turn out to be rotten and terrible? Let's clear those points of view.

> *All the decisions, judgments, compilations, and conclusions that you have to be the perfect mother, the perfect father, the perfect sister, the perfect brother, the perfect child, the perfect aunt, the perfect uncle, the perfect example, the perfect teacher, the perfect nanny, the perfect grandparent, and that you have to show that you are the perfect son or daughter by raising your children just like your parents raised you, will you now destroy and uncreate it all? Right and Wrong, Good and Bad, POD and POC, All 9, Shorts, Boys, and Beyonds.*

20

GRATITUDE, LOVE, AND CARING

*What if your greatest potency is the gentleness that you can be, the
kindness you can be, the caring you are, and the space of
infinite allowance you be?*
~ Dr. Dain Heer

Gary:

My friend, Annie, who has a horse ranch, says that sometimes people visit her ranch to be with the horses and to hug them. Some of
these people will walk up to a horse as if they are charging it because
they want something from it. The horse looks at them and asks,
"Who are you?" It won't have anything to do with them. The people
are crushed.

These people aren't there to give anything to the horse. They don't
see the horse that's in front of them, they don't ask what the horse
might desire or require from them, they don't find out what they can
gift to the horse; they are simply there to receive. If they paid attention to the horse and knew how to do it, the horse would gift them
with attention. But from the horse's point of view (and from mine
too), their behavior doesn't communicate caring in any way.

This is yet another thing we've learned from the animal world. When
you are grateful for the horse or the dog or the cat exactly the way he
or she is, everything works. You can freely gift to them and receive

from them. The same is true for your kids. How do you show your children you care for them? You show them you are grateful for them.

Gratitude is tangible to a child; love is intangible. Love is confusing. There are too many definitions for *love*.

Anne:

There are as many definitions and manifestations of *love* as there are people. Take, for example, the phrase, "I love you." What does that mean to you? Probably not the same thing it means to me. I often hear parents say to their kids, either directly or indirectly, "If you loved me you would ____." That love is conditional on the child being and/or doing what the parent wants. In angry homes or homes where there is violence, love is coupled with threats, fear, and/or physical harm. Parents say things like "I'm doing this because I love you." In other relationships, love and guilt go hand-in-hand. In one family I know about, the child was blamed by his parents for their financial situation: "If we hadn't had you, we'd have more money." In some families, love is contingent on performance—grades, income, achievements, or applause. In all of these examples, love comes with judgment attached.

Gary:

Communicating a sense of gratitude is far more important than telling the child you love him or her. I talked with a man in Australia whose ex-wife had taken their daughter out of the country. He hadn't seen the girl for seventeen months. She was about to return, and he was unsure about how to approach her. He asked me how he could rekindle their connection.

I said, "Your daughter has been away from you for a long time, but have you ever truly lost the connection with her?"

"No," he replied. He realized that the connection had not been lost, even though they hadn't been together in over a year.

I said, "Sometimes the parent who takes a child away tries to make leaving okay with the child by saying things like 'Your father doesn't want you.' Ask your daughter questions like 'Are you aware that I searched for you this whole time? What were you told about my point of view? Are you aware that you are the most important thing in my life? Are you aware that I care about you so much and that I am grateful to have you in my life?' Then say, 'Thank you so much for coming back to me.'"

In this reality, love is about judgment and criticism. Gratitude is not. Gratitude is the place in which you are grateful to the person for showing up in your life, grateful for having them any time that you have them, with no judgment. Unlike love, gratitude can only exist without judgment.

The first step is to have gratitude for you. When you don't have gratitude for you, you can't have it for your child. And if you don't have gratitude, you have to judge. Be grateful for the things you're able to accomplish in life, be grateful for the things you're able to perceive in life, and be grateful for the fact that you don't have to judge you. Once you do that, you can start being in allowance of you—and everyone else around you, especially your child.

Anne:

What if you could have gratitude for your child just the way he or she is, regardless of what others think, in spite of what others say? What if you could embrace your child's differences?

Kids with autism function primarily from energy rather than emotions, thoughts, or feelings. They show affection very differently from other kids; in fact, sometimes there may be no physical evidence of affection or love, because often they dislike cuddling, hugging, or making eye contact. However, if you tune into your child energetically, you'll know what's going on in their world.

When Temple Grandin was asked during a TEDx Talk whether it might be unrealistic for the parents of an autistic child to think that their child loves them, she responded, "Well, let me tell you, your child will be loyal, and if the house is burning down, they're going to get you out of it."

A five-year-old boy who was on the autism spectrum was brought to see me because he had stopped speaking. He made no eye contact with me and had his dad speak and get toys for him. In the first session, I sat on the floor and spoke with his dad. I kept the boy in my peripheral vision because I knew that if I looked at him directly, it would be too much for him. I simply made myself available to him energetically. I made no demands on him at all. By the end of the first session, he was playing with toys on the floor, sitting close to me with his back turned to me.

At the end of three months, he was speaking, not only to me but also to his parents and to people in the community. Did he like me? Yes. Did I like him? Yes. Did we show affection by hugging or physical touch? No. How could I tell he liked me? By the way his eyes would light up as he caught sight of me in the reception room, the way he insisted on telling me stories and shushed his dad when Dad tried to clarify things, and the way he said to his dad, "Dad, we live here now. We don't have to go home!"

His dad understood all of that and did not place demands on him to be cuddly like his younger brother. Nor did he require his son to be someone he wasn't; instead, he demonstrated his caring by facilitating his son in learning tools so he could function with more ease in the world.

Gary says, "True caring is when you don't defend anyone or anything." This boy's dad was not defending his son, nor was he defending anyone's point of view. He was simply in allowance—grateful for his son just as he was.

Gary:

For me, true caring is about being in allowance and acknowledging the infinite choice that kids have. True caring is when you allow the other person to be exactly who they are and to do exactly what they do, and you have no point of view about it.

21

THE ABILITY AND WILLINGNESS TO PERCEIVE WHAT IS

If kids pick up the thoughts, feelings, and emotions of the people all around them, and you project on them that they're disabled, what have you done?

~ Gary Douglas

Gary:

Perceiving means being aware of what's currently occurring. When you perceive something, you have the awareness of what is here right now, without reaching the conclusion that therefore it will be like that forever. What shows up tomorrow may be different. When you perceive what is and you ask a question instead of reaching a conclusion, you will have even greater awareness.

Anne:

In the previous chapter, I talked about a five-year-old boy on the autism spectrum who had stopped speaking. When his dad first brought him to my office, the boy refused to speak, let alone acknowledge my presence. If I had turned my perception of him into the conclusion that something was wrong with him or that he would never speak again, I would have sent him the energy that he was already receiving from many different sources. I would have been like the mother Dain mentioned who was researching the symptoms of autism on the Internet, and whose son, Nicolas, picked them up out of her head and began to exhibit those symptoms and behaviors.

However, instead of drawing conclusions about my client who wasn't speaking, I asked questions, like:

- What is this?
- What would it take for this to change?
- What's right about this I'm not getting?
- What's he telling us (by speaking only selectively)?
- What's the value of not speaking?

Those questions gave me huge awareness of the boy, his family, and what was possible for him. They also gave me other questions to ask him and his Dad so they could have greater awareness.

Perceiving is not about pretending that something that is, isn't. It's not about saying, "It's all good," when in fact there may be stuff going on that isn't working and could be changed. It's not blind faith that somehow, if you just think positive thoughts, everything will work out in the end. No! It's about being willing to be with what is. In the case of this little boy, it was about perceiving that he was not talking and then asking questions about what would it take for that to change.

The Willingness to See What Is
Gary:

The key to considering new possibilities for yourself and your child is the ability and willingness to see what is. The willingness to see what is—to perceive it and receive it—is the essential factor. Without this ability, parents won't be able to receive the information they need and they won't be able to see what's possible with their child. They will function, as so many people do, from their previously-made decisions, conclusions, and judgments rather than a clear sense of the extraordinary being who is in front of them.

Dain:

If you do not have total access to perceiving something, it's because somewhere along the line, you decided it wasn't possible. For example, if you have decided that there is no way you can perceive everything that is going on in an autistic kid's universe, including all the information they're communicating and receiving, then there is no way you'll ever be able to perceive that.

Anne:

As a parent, what if, every morning, you could destroy and uncreate anywhere you are unwilling to perceive and receive *what is* regarding your child?

> *Anywhere I am unwilling to perceive and receive what is regarding my child, I destroy and uncreate it all. Right and Wrong, Good and Bad, POD and POC, All 9, Shorts, Boys, and Beyonds.*

Gary:

Sometimes parents may begin to perceive the truth of their kids, which is great, but at the same time, they want their child to fit into all the norms and expectations of this reality. They're stuck in a fixed point of view about how that's supposed to look. They will acknowledge that yes, they see their child's talents and abilities, and they are sincere in this, and then they'll ask, "So, how do we get him to be normal? How do we get him to fit in?"

Dain:

That would be like Einstein's mom asking, "How do I get Albert to forget this theory of relativity he is working on and become a little more normal?"

Gary:

Yeah, "Albert, just do regular math. Don't do that weird stuff." It's as if we are attempting to turn the Einsteins of the world into bean counters. It is not possible; it cannot work that way, but we keep trying, as though somehow it's going to work.

Dain:

It seems that no one is looking at this from the point of view of "What's possible here?" Instead everybody is saying, "You're screwed up. How do we make you normal? How do we diminish your capacity so that you'll fit in with us?" It's like we have people who can fly but we want to stop that. We buy them lead boots, and if it turns out that they are really powerful flyers even with the lead boots on, we buy them lead suits.

Gary:

In the United States, we have adopted an assembly-line, mass-production point of view. We stamp out a product and make it over and over again. We have mass-produced food and restaurants. You can go to a MacDonald's, Kentucky Fried Chicken, or Pizza Hut anywhere in the world and get the same product. Whatever it is, they make everything the same. The necessity of making everything the same has taken away the value of individuality.

We all learn uniquely, and unfortunately, the idea of being unique and learning uniquely has gone out of fashion. We favor the cookie-cutter approach now. And we're on a destruction course. We are consuming the planet as rapidly as possible, which is why the X-Men may have something very important to tell us about how *not* being normal is a very good thing.

Dain and I spent some time with a young, autistic boy in Perth who had an amazing ability to work with clay. He would form beautiful, huge dinosaurs in about three minutes. His mother had come to us because she was having a terrible time with him. She wanted him to be more "normal."

Dain:

We said to the mother, "He's so bright!"

Gary:

The mother said, "But he's not speaking."

I asked, "Does he need to speak for you to know what he is doing?"

She said, "Well, no, but he has to speak in order to go to school."

I said, "Well, maybe so at the moment, but hopefully there will come a time when that is not a necessity."

After we worked with this little boy, he looked at us directly in the eyes. He was saying, "Thanks, thanks, thanks."

Then he crawled up in his mother's lap and hugged her. She burst into tears because this eight-year-old kid had never before crawled into her lap and cuddled with her. It was a huge change.

It was unfortunate that his mother was so focused on his learning to function in a linear way, because with his artistic capacity, the boy could be an extraordinary artist. Regrettably, his artistic capacity will never be developed because instead of seeing what he can do, his parents and teachers are trying to develop his linear abilities so he's more like everyone else. They don't value the difference he is; they're actually afraid of it. A huge part of our school systems is afraid of things that are different.

Parents With a Vested Interest in Having a "Disabled" Child

I had a girl in one of my classes in New York who had paranoid schizophrenia. She was a portal, a point of entry for entities. During the class, we closed down the portals, and the entities who were hanging around moved away from her. It made her life much easier.

A few days later, I went to lunch with the girl's psychiatrist and her parents. The psychiatrist wanted to know what I had done because I had gotten a result in a weekend that he couldn't get in a lifetime.

I said, "We just closed down the portals and taught her to deal with entities."

The girl's mother turned to me and said, "No, it's not what *you* did." Then she turned to the psychiatrist and stated, "It's the drugs you gave her. You finally got the right medications."

The psychiatrist looked at her and thought, "Oh, now I know what the problem is."

I knew what the problem was too. The mother wanted her daughter disabled; she didn't want her child to be able to handle her own life.

Parents like this mother can become upset when you take away their kids' so-called disabilities. They want to prove how much they care for their kids by showing how special their kids are. There is something valuable for them in sticking their child with a label. It gives them someone who will never leave them. They have the kid forever that way. And they don't want to acknowledge that they could have a different possibility.

What's going on in cases like these, where parents are invested in having their X-Man child be "normal" or "special" rather than who they actually are? They are not perceiving, seeing, or receiving the incredible being who is in front of them. They're finding a wrongness in their child that they are either resisting and reacting to—or aligning and agreeing with. But what if there's no wrongness to begin with?

I worked with a little kid in Perth who touched furniture all the time. He had been taken to many shrinks, psychologists, and people who tested and evaluated him. I sat down with him and said, "I'm not here to test you. I'm not here to do anything but talk to you about what you can do and how there is nothing wrong with you."

He was not into having that conversation. He sat with me for a while and then he reached out to touch the furniture. I watched him for a few minutes and asked, "What information do you get from the furniture when you touch it?"

No one had ever recognized that. The boy went, "Wah! This guy is getting something different from everybody else!"

I asked, "Do you realize that you are like Harry Potter? You have magic in you that you can touch things and they talk to you."

The boy thought a moment and said, "Yeah, I am like that."

Dain:

Everyone else made his abilities a wrongness. Can you imagine what it would be like for you if you had an amazing ability and everybody saw you as weird, disabled, and wrong? How would you end up going through your life? Would you expand into your abilities—or would you shut them off as much as possible?

After that, the boy was able to let go of some of his considerations that he was disabled. It's truly unfortunate that so many kids who have the abilities we've described are called disabled.

Gary:

Is it helpful to a child when people see him or her as disabled or dysfunctional? No! These children are in unnecessary pain and suffering because we keep trying to make them finite rather than seeing what their true capacities are. We project on them that they are disabled, stupid, wrong, and different from everybody else. They pick up all that stuff, even if it's not said out loud.

Somebody tells kids they are disabled, and then they try to become what they are told they are. Got the name, play the game. A teacher told me that she had kids in her classroom who were told they had ADD. It was clear to her that these kids did not have ADD; they had begun to mimic the behavior of other kids who did have it. She said to me, "This is a huge problem. How would you deal with it?"

I said, "Diagnosis is deadly. If you can show kids that you don't see their abilities as disabilities, it can make a huge difference for them. One thing you can do upfront is ask the kids if they are really disabled—or whether they have an ability." They often know they have extraordinary abilities, and asking the question allows them to know what they know.

In the final analysis, acknowledging that kids—all kids—are infinite beings with an infinite ability to perceive, know, be, and receive is the single most important thing that you, as a parent or teacher, can do to assist them. This is especially true for kids with autism, OCD, ADD, ADHD and all those other labels, because truly, they have special gifts.

Anne:

I have worked with many parents who bought into the labels and diagnoses placed on their children, not because they necessarily believed in them, but because they were not aware that there was another way of looking at all of that. They were functioning from the space of doing the best they could with the information that was available to them at the time. Even those who seemed to behave as if they needed their child to have a problem or a disability sometimes changed their way of operating when another possibility was presented to them. I am willing to hang in there with parents who keep coming back to see me, even if there does not seem to be much change in the moment. The ones who are wedded to the notion that their child has something wrong with them are the ones who stop coming into see me, not because I drive them away, but because I

Separation or Integration?

Gary:

I've been asked whether it's best for X-Men kids to be integrated with so-called normal kids in school—or whether it's better for them to be in classrooms with kids who are more like they are. My perspective is that it is probably most helpful to separate them and give them tools for dealing with the world and understanding that they have abilities—not disabilities. Then they can be integrated with the other kids, as they are willing to be integrated. If you ask them, they'll tell you when they want to be integrated.

Dain:

It may be easier for younger kids to be integrated with other kids in classrooms because the younger kids don't know what "disabled" means, so they don't project that label as heavily onto themselves; however, they will begin to do that if teachers and parents are doing it.

Gary:

Some of the kids we've heard about have chosen to be integrated. Initially they didn't wish to be in classes with the other kids because they didn't like dealing with kids who saw them as "disabled."

Their teacher said, "Hey, you're more like Harry Potter; you're more like the X-Men."

They said, "I am?"

She said, "Yeah, you're a mutant."

The kids said, "Oh, okay, great." It was okay with them to be a mutant, because the kids in the X-Men movies are totally cool and don't function like other people. That little twist made it possible for them to be with the other kids even if the other kids made fun of them for being "special."

don't take the position that there is anything wrong with their child or with them.

How do I work with each parent? I always ask them what they would like to get out of having me as the therapist for their child. And I don't take a position on whatever it is that they say. I ask them lots of questions, and many of them are able to shift into a different space regarding their child. And some choose not to. Some shift quickly; others take lots of time. I had a mother thank me recently for not judging her for being so reluctant to change and for being patient with her. As Gary says, "You hears it when you hears it!"

~ 22 ~

THE LANGUAGE OF ENERGY

The primary language of life is energy.
- Gary Douglas

Anne:

One of the first questions I remember hearing from an Access Consciousness facilitator was, "What if your first language was energy?" Now, that made sense to me! I had always wondered how, as a child of four, I had been able to comfort crying babies without saying a word. What if it was the language of energy we were speaking?

When your children were babies, could you tell the difference between a tired-cry, a wet-diaper-cry, and a hungry-cry? Before your child's vocabulary was developed, were you able to know what he or she needed? Were you able to communicate? That is what I call the language of energy. It's not verbal and it's certainly not cognitive. The language of energy bypasses your logical brain and goes to what's underneath that's actually the heart of what's being communicated.

Following the death of my stepfather, my mom lived with my husband and me for the last two years of her life. She had profound dementia, and over time, both her short-term and long-term memory were affected. She had three favorite questions she would ask, as if they were loops: "What time is it?" "What's the date?" and "Where's Josie?" (Josie was her cat.) And from the time the answer left your lips, she couldn't remember your response—ever.

Periodically, she would become upset and say things like, "Why am I still alive? I've lived too long! I don't want to be around anymore!" I asked the hospice chaplain what I could say to my mom that could soothe her, and he described what he referred to as "conversations of the heart." From my perspective, these conversations had less to do with the heart and more to do with communicating with energy.

So, I said to her, "I don't know why you're still here either, Mama. I'm glad that you are. I don't want you to go a minute sooner than you would like to go or stay a minute longer than you would like to be here. You'll know when it's time, and I'll do whatever I can to assist you." And because she was my mom, I reassured her that I was happy, that I would never forget her, and that I was so grateful to her. I thanked her for everything she had done for me.

Her relief was visible. Her body relaxed, the worries disappeared from her face, and she did not ask that question again for several months. And when she did ask it again, I said the same things, with the same results, until she chose to leave.

Even though I used words to speak with her, it was clear to me that what she received was the energy of my communication—not unlike the crying babies I had been able to soothe as a young child.

Dain:

Have you ever given someone a hug and felt like you could stand there forever, melting, falling into the person you were hugging? And, by contrast, have you ever given someone a hug where it felt like you were hugging a rock on legs? Are these two experiences different? Then you know what we mean when we talk about energy.

These are two totally different energetic experiences—two totally different "energies."

It is that simple.

Gary:

What is the basis of the universe? Energy. Every particle of the universe has energy and consciousness. Energy is the substance by which transformation occurs. Energy is present, mutable, and changeable upon request.

You give and receive much more communication energetically than you do with words, but if you are like most people, you are largely unaware of what you're communicating with energy. We're looking to see if we can open the communications you have with your kids, so you can communicate on an energetic level. Anne does this all the time in her work. When she's in a session with kids, sometimes she uses pictures to communicate and sometimes she doesn't use pictures—but it's never just a linear communication using words. It's always an instantaneous energetic communication that goes from her to the kid. It's "What are you doing? I'm here. I'm here with you."

Autistic kids excel at communicating energetically. This is one of the areas where we are far less aware than they are. These kids have an intense awareness of the energies in a room. It is far more intense than most of us can handle.

Dain:

If your kid is not verbal, just acknowledge where he or she functions from.

Anne:

And acknowledge what he or she is picking up on. For example, if there are financial worries or worries about a grandparent, pretending those things are not occurring is a mistake. Kids are far more able to tap into the energy of what's going on than most of us give them credit for. Even if your child is not verbal, you can speak to him or her as I did to my mom, and your child will get it. You certainly don't need to share unnecessary details with your child, but by acknowledging the energy of what's going on, you give your child the gift of his or her awareness.

Gary:

Kids get that, especially kids with autism. When the energy of a situation doesn't match the words that are spoken, they become confused and may respond in a variety of ways, from becoming extremely agitated to shutting down and checking out. For them, the world is an insane place where what people think isn't what comes out of their mouth and what people think doesn't match what they do.

Autistic kids feel all that, but they can't make sense of it. They can't create any order in their universe about it. When you start to talk about these things with them, the chaos in their universe begins to straighten out. They start to realize, "Oh, I don't have to do anything about that. It doesn't really matter." When they get that there is somebody they can link with and communicate with, it starts to create a sense of peace in them. A lot of their edginess starts to go away.

Dain:

If your kid is not verbal, just acknowledge where he or she functions from. If you're the parent or the teacher of an autistic child or somebody who interacts with autistic kids, you can say, "Hey, you know what? Communicating with energy is an ability. Hardly anybody understands this. We can practice how you're going to be able to communicate with the outside world." You provide a way for them to actually begin to communicate with the rest of the world.

An Experiment

A friend of mine who works with special needs kids in the public school system told me about an "experiment" she did, connecting with kids in their own space. She wanted to play with energetic communication to see if it really worked.

She decided that she was not going to speak to the kids when she went in to the classroom to work with some of the students. She wouldn't try to make eye contact with them. She would just go from the front of the classroom to the back of the room, where the computers were, and she would sit at one of the computers. Her idea was to see if she could connect energetically with the kids without using words, eye contact, or body language.

So, she sat in the back of the room at a computer and just asked to be space and to connect with the kids. In less than thirty seconds, a young student who was about ten feet away, turned around, looked at her dead in the eye and said, "I love you."

My friend said, "I was willing to go out to where he was and to just be the space, and that became an invitation for him to connect with me."

Anne:

When I talk about communicating with energy, many people I speak with tell me they can't communicate this way. What if that is not true? In fact, even if we're not aware of it, isn't that primarily how we do communicate?

Take, for example, a time at home that might be fraught with drama and upset, such as getting out of the house on time in the morning. What happens energetically in your home when the first alarm clock goes off? Then the next one? Then when it's time to wake up your child, who would prefer not to leave bed or home? And on and on…Isn't there an energetic pattern that has been established that translates into *mornings are awful?* Can you feel the energy going between all the members of your household, the energy of *here we go again?*

Also, take as an example a time with your child that was sweet, easy, and joyful, like playing in a lake or a swimming pool, reading a book together, or just being in the same room together peacefully. Can you tap into the energy of that? Do you see how you were communicating energetically with one another?

TIPS AND TOOLS FOR
SUCCEEDING IN SCHOOL

"Give me the answer."
We are entrained from the time we go to school to have the answer.
~ Gary Douglas

Anne:

Currently, the education system functions from a mentality of "learn this, repeat this, parrot it back, learn this, repeat this, parrot it back." Is that learning—or is that programming? Basically the schools are programming children to be good citizens; it's training them to work well with the rest of the world and not make waves.

One of the targets we have with Access Consciousness is getting schools together that will help all kids tap into their knowing. We have run into a number of students, even in the regular school system, who have the ability to instantly know the answer to a math question—but they can't show the steps of how they got to the answer; in fact, those steps don't exist for them because they simply *know* the answer. This can also happen in science or any other area. The kid looks at a problem or a question and bam!—he or she has the answer.

Teachers tend to make kids wrong for this. As a result, the kids often think there is something wrong with them because they *knew*—but couldn't prove their answer or tell how they arrived at it. If we, as parents, teachers, and educators, can get to the point where we recognize that we, as beings, can function from our knowing in this way, we can change the whole education system.

Tool: Are You Getting the Answer as Soon as the Question Is Asked?

Dain:

If you have a child who has problems in science, math, or any other area where he or she has to provide answers to questions, the first thing to ask the child is "Are you getting the answer to the question as soon as the question is asked or as soon as you read it?"

At one point, Gary's youngest daughter was getting C's and D's in science and math. She asked, "Will you tutor me?"

I thought, "Are you kidding me?" I had no idea how to tutor somebody, but I said, "Okay, we will see how this works."

We sat down together and I said, "Do some of these problems for me. Let me see where your head goes and what's going on." I saw that as soon as she read a question, an answer would pop into her head. I could feel it energetically. She would read, read, read and be in the question mode and all of a sudden there would be a little energetic "pop" when she'd get the answer. But instead of trusting her knowing, she would then try to figure out the answer, because nobody ever said, "Hey, you can have an answer just pop into your head. It's okay."

So, instead of going with the answer she *knew*, she would try to *figure out* an answer—and she would get it wrong most of the time. She already had the answer, but she didn't trust it. It was amazing to see this in action.

I had her read the question and I would stop her as soon as I could see that the answer came up. I would say, "Okay stop! What did you get? Write it down." She would write the answer down, and it would always be the correct answer or part of it. It happened instantaneously—but then she would try to figure out or "prove" it, and that's where she got into trouble.

She was feeling dumb and hopeless; she thought she didn't know anything about the subjects she was studying, but once she saw that she actually had the answers, she realized she actually knew a lot.

Expanding Out

Anne:

During the school day, typically kids are asked to pay attention and to focus, which means they have to contract their universe as well as their awareness. When this happens, events can take on a significance, importance, or density that result in upsets and discomfort. For example, when a slow math teacher doesn't understand how a high-speed X-Man kid did a math problem, the X-Man kid may believe the math teacher thinks he is stupid and wrong, and he may then get upset or withdraw.

I might ask the kid to expand out by being aware that the math teacher is slow and he is lightening fast. When kids expand out, the things that are going on around them become less significant and they gain awareness and clarity about what is. They lose the heaviness and contraction of judgment and wrongness, and they become space. So, the kid would see that he is not wrong and the math teacher is not wrong; the two of them just think and communicate differently. The kid gets that he does not need to change who he is and that maybe he can explain in language the math teacher gets, the steps he took that got him to the correct math answer.

Working Through the Problem Backwards

Often the best way to do this is to work through the problem backwards or in a non-linear way. Ask the child to start with the answer, and move backwards towards the beginning of the math problem. Oftentimes, that's enough of a shift for them to find words to describe to the teacher how they arrived at the answer. X-Men kids don't go from point A to points B, C, and D in that order. They tell me that they get a little bit here, then another little bit there. It's out of sequence from this reality's perspective, yet it makes complete sense to them—and their answers are correct. Of course, it takes a math teacher who is willing to step beyond the rules of how math is supposed to be taught and learned. When teachers are willing to listen and see what is, they often get it.

Tool: What's Your First Language?

Gary:

I worked with an American kid who had spoken English his whole life. He was going to a Jewish school and was studying English and Hebrew. He was getting A's in Hebrew and spoke it like a native, and he was failing his English class. He couldn't seem to comprehend what was going on.

I asked him "What's your first language?" Asking this question is a way to invite people to the awareness of what their first language is. Sometimes the correct response is that their first language is energy. Other times, when a person is blocked from accessing a specific language, the question invites them to have the awareness of what their first spoken language was.

He said, "Hebrew."

We destroyed and uncreated everything that did not allow English to be like a first language to him—not a first language, but *like* a first language, where he knew all the lifetimes in which he had all that information available.

We also destroyed and uncreated all the lifetimes in which he had known English and had been able to write English and to speak it fluently, including all he times he had been a professor of English. This allowed him to clear all his decisions, judgments, conclusions, and fixed points of view about speaking and writing English from those lifetimes. And finally, we destroyed and uncreated everything that kept him from knowing that he could speak and write in English as well as he could in Hebrew. Almost instantly, he shifted and started getting A's in English.

Tool: Destroy and Uncreate Everything That....

You can also teach kids to destroy and uncreate anything that doesn't allow them to read at 300 words per minute and retain everything they've read—or everything that doesn't allow them to perceive, know, be, and receive the totality of what's on every page instantaneously—or everything that doesn't allow them to know the answers to the test right up front. You can ask your kids to say:

> *Everything that doesn't allow me to read at 300 words per minute and retain everything I've read, I destroy and uncreate it all. Right and Wrong, Good and Bad, POD and POC, All 9, Shorts, Boys, and Beyonds.*

Tool: Going into the Teacher's Head

When kids are studying for a test, let them know that they can pick the answer out of their teacher's head. Say, "When you take a test, go into the teacher's head and ask which answer is right according to the teacher. You can take the answer out of the teacher's head."

I have had kids do this, and they call me up and they say, "Thanks, Gary. I got an A on my test."

I say, "Good!" I know one young lady who is getting straight A's in junior college because she picks the answers out of her teachers' heads. When she has to write an essay she says, "Okay, everything that the teacher wants me to know, that I know, let me have that information." She starts writing without thinking about what she's writing and she gets A's on every exam. This is an ability we all have. We all have the ability to know. We might as well use it.

When you acknowledge kids' talents and their ability to know, they can perform more easily in school. They're willing to say, "Okay, I'm going to take the answer out of people's heads. I'll know this and I'll know that."

Dain:

I have to say that I thought Gary was full of crap when I first heard this. I had studied hard in school and I graduated with honors. When I heard Gary talk about our ability to pick information out of other people's heads, my attitude was "Come on! No way, man. You can't do this!"

Then I started talking to some of the kids in Access Consciousness. I asked, "Have you tried this stuff?"

They said, "Yeah."

I asked, "Well, does it work?"

They said, "Yeah, and school is so much easier."

I asked, "Are you still learning stuff?"

They said, "Yeah, actually I am learning more."

I asked, "Really? How are you learning more?"

Gary:

They said things like "I don't have to try to remember it" and "I don't have to try to shove the material in and I don't get frantic before a test because I always know I'm going to have the answer."

Are you one of those people who did the "burning the midnight oil" version of studying? How did that work for you? Do you remember and use any of that information?

Dain:

I was a business economics major when I went to the university because it was the easiest major I could find. In one of my truly boring economics classes, I only went to class three times; for the first day of class, the midterm exam, and the final. Without realizing it, I did exactly what Gary is talking about. When I studied the course materials I would ask, "What would the professor want me to know about this?" There were three concepts out of an entire semester of material that he wanted everybody to know, and I happened to get those three things.

Gary:

You *happened* to get those three things?

Dain:

Weird, huh?

Gary:

No, it's not weird. You got those concepts because you asked the question, "What would the professor want me to know about this?"

Teach your kids to ask a question that's going to give them the awareness of what they need to study—not to study everything, thinking they are going to fail if they don't get the answer that is needed.

Tool: What Do I Have to Know Here, in Order to Pass the Test?

Here's another tool you can teach kids when they are reading their textbooks: What do I have to know here, in order to pass the test? When you use this tool, as you read, all of a sudden, your eyes will focus on the thing you need to know, and you'll say, "Okay! That's the thing I will remember."

Dain:

Just ask that one question, "What am I going to have to know here?" As you read the material, your brain will pick out and store the information you'll need to pass the test. That's the way your brain works. You ask a question and your brain says, "Hey, I'm here to deliver."

Gary:

When you, the being, ask the question, you will be able to know exactly what you need to know.

Dain:

It's part of that "Ask and you shall receive" thing.

Tool: What Is It the Teacher Wants Me to Put in This Paper?

Gary:

I talked with a mother whose daughter has ADHD. The girl had an assignment to write a paper, and she had written it in her head, but she couldn't get it down on a sheet of paper.

I said to the mother, "Have your daughter ask: What is it the teacher wants me to put in this paper? Tell her to ask that question and then let go of her point of view and just start to write. She'll find out that she knows a whole lot more than she thinks she knows, and it will all be there. It will get easy."

Dain:

This is a very helpful tool for kids who are having trouble writing a paper. They may have to repeat the question a few times as they write, but each time they ask, the process of writing will get easier.

Gary:

You can also cheat by tapping into the teacher's head and asking what the teacher knows that you can know.

Dain:

When we say, "Cheat in school" we mean cheat from awareness. Don't cheat from unawareness.

Gary:

Don't copy from someone else's work, because if you do that, you are going to get the wrong answer. Instead ask what the teacher knows that you need to put down. Or ask, "What is the answer that all the kids who know the right answer are giving?"

If a kid with OCD has a friend in the classroom and that friend is on his wavelength, the kid with OCD will write down the same answer his friend did, even if it's wrong. This happens all the time. And then of course, if they are sitting next to each other, they'll get accused of cheating. But it's not cheating.

I was talking with the younger brother of the boy who excelled in Hebrew but did less well in English. The brother had recently started Hebrew school and he was having trouble with it. I said, "All you have to do is think of your brother, and the Hebrew words will come."

I also gave him a process he could do:

> *Everything that does not allow me to pick up all the Hebrew that my brother knows without having to read it, and every-*

*thing that does not allow me to tap into his brain to get the
information I desire, I destroy and uncreate all of that. Right
and Wrong, Good and Bad, POD and POC, All 9, Shorts,
Boys, and Beyonds.*

Reading to Kids

Reading aloud to kids is a great way of increasing their fluency. When
you read books with autistic children, they'll start to speak and read
in a different way. However, the way we read to them now is too
slow for them. You can't read a book to them word by word. You
have to give them a download of the whole page and flip through
the pages very quickly.

In other words, you read the book with the awareness that you have
the ability to *think* all the sounds on the page. Have you ever noticed
that you can think faster than you can speak? That's what I'm talking
about. When you're reading to your child, just think that you are
saying all the words on the page out loud and turn the pages just a
little slower than your child would do it (which is usually very fast).
It's as though you are reading to him without speaking. Give the
child the picture and the words at exactly the same time. This is the
way to begin to open the doors for communication to begin.

I suggested this to a mother whose eight-year-old barely spoke.

Three weeks later, she called me and said, "My son is reading. More
than that, he's speaking in complete sentences for the first time in
his entire life."

All she did was turn the pages of the book at the same rate he did,
while giving him a download of what it would sound like if she was
reading it aloud but as fast as he would get it. Boom! Boom! Boom!
He was doing full sentences in eight weeks.

Have you ever done a speed-reading course? The target is to get
you to read the whole page at once so that you literally flip through

the pages and see everything that is on the pages. At the end of the book or the chapter, you'll know everything about it. That's the way autistic kids do it.

In these speed-reading courses, they start out by moving you down the page very slowly, so do that. Then increase your speed as you get the hang of it. Or you might want to play with reading the book backwards, going page by page backwards and see what happens. There are lots of different things you can play with to see what the results could be. We need to do some more research into this approach as we have only had the opportunity to work on it with a few kids.

Anne:

An adult friend of ours told us recently that she was never able to read from left to right or top to bottom. She said, "Instead I receive the energy of the words I need to have my eyes see. They pop off the page and they literally make themselves known to me."

Gary told her, "It's all the things you need to know. What if you asked yourself, 'What does this page tell me?'"

I know that what we talk about here may sound odd or "out there." Guess what? It is! And, guess what else? It really works! Even though you may not be comfortable with some or all of any of this, try doing something different. You might be surprised at the changes you and your child create.

~ 24 ~

WE ALL HAVE THE ABILITIES THE
X-MEN HAVE

*The X-Men and their abilities have been our focus, but these are
places that you function from as well. We all have these abilities, but
when we don't acknowledge them, we create a limitation of ourselves. We try to linearize ourselves into the normalcy of this reality.*

~ Gary Douglas

Gary:

The X-Men and their abilities have been our focus in this book, and
we have talked about them at length, but we want to emphasize that
these are capabilities you have as well, even though you may not
realize it yet. We all have the abilities they have. You may have a lot
of fixed points of view about things you think you can't do anything
about. Well, we're here to tell you can do something about those
things.

> *How many decisions, judgments, and conclusions do you have
> about what ADD, ADHD, autism, and OCD are? Have you
> concluded they are a bad thing or a limitation? Or that there
> is no solution to them? Everything that is, will you destroy and
> uncreate it so you can see a different possibility, please? Right
> and Wrong, Good and Bad, POD and POC, All 9, Shorts,
> Boys, and Beyonds.*

Anne:

If you are reading this book, chances are that you have talents, abilities, and awareness that extend far beyond the capacity of your cognitive mind.

What if you are way more psychic and aware than you give yourself credit for?

How many times have you thought about someone, and then that person called you or sent you an email? Or you saw them and said, "Oh, I was just thinking about you!"

How many times have you known exactly what someone was about to say before they said it?

Do you think faster than you can speak?

Have you ever known ahead of time what was going to happen, and then it did?

Have you ever asked the universe to assist you in getting the money together for something you really wanted to do or to have—and it did?

When you were in school, did your teachers write on your report cards, "Doesn't live up to her full potential" or "Doesn't finish what he starts" or "Has difficulty focusing and concentrating" or "Is impulsive—blurts out"?

Has anyone ever called you weird?

Have you tried desperately to fit in and then given up and resigned yourself to a life of being the one who laughs at the wrong time, makes the comment that silences a group, and dresses "inappropriately" (even though it turns out that you are the envy of everyone who had wanted to dress like you but didn't have the courage to do it)?

Do you judge yourself unrelentingly for being so different?

Do you go crazy from boredom unless you are in motion, learning new things, and creating beyond what's deemed acceptable?

How many books are you reading at the same time?

What if there's nothing wrong with you? What if different is just different—not wrong? Is there a way you can use that difference to your advantage? What would that look like?

Do you ever wonder why people say one thing when they so clearly mean another?

Do you ever wonder how some people can be so mean and get away with it? And what about the kind ones, who are so badly treated?

Do you ever feel as if your head will explode from all the craziness you see, that everyone seems to think is normal?

Have you ever been able sit still? Ever?

Have you ever been able to make your mind slow down? Ever?

Have you ever been able to make your mind have just one thought at a time? Ever?

Have you always had the magic touch with animals or kids? Are you the one they know has their back?

If you are a teacher or work in the school system, are you the one the kids look forward to seeing?

Whether you are a parent or not, are you the one the kids are drawn to?

Have you always known something else was possible, yet not known *what* or *how*?

Here are some tools you can use to tap into what you do know:

Tool: Energy, Space and Consciousness
Ask:

> *What energy, space and consciousness can my body and I be that will allow us to be the energy, space and consciousness we truly be in school, at home, with the kids, at work, or wherever we are? Everything that doesn't allow that, I destroy and uncreate it all. Right and Wrong, Good and Bad, POD and POC, All 9, Shorts, Boys, and Beyonds.*

My friend Trina asks this question before entering a classroom. She says that no matter how chaotic and agitated the kids are, within a minute or two, the kids calm down and the classroom becomes more peaceful.

Tool: Get out of Judgment
Every time you find yourself judging yourself or having a point of view about what someone else should or should not do, POD and POC it all. Say:

> *Everything this is, I destroy and uncreate it all. Right and Wrong, Good and Bad, POD and POC, All 9, Shorts, Boys, and Beyonds.*

You don't have to define what "this" is. You have the energy of the density of limitation, and without labeling it, you can destroy and uncreate it all.

Tool: Choose
Your choices don't have to last forever. If you make a choice and it doesn't work out, you can choose something else. For example,

if you choose to take your child to the movie and it soon becomes clear that he or she will not be able to sit through it, you can choose something else. If you find yourself angry or frightened, you can make another choice, such as asking a question like, "Who does this belong to?" or using the clearing statement.

Tool: What Am I Aware Of?

Ask: What am I aware of that I'm not acknowledging? It is a wonderful question to ask when you feel sad, worried, or angry.

Tool: What Do I Know?

When you start to think, analyze, look for answers, or try to figure things out, ask: What do I know that I'm pretending not to know? You might be surprised at what comes up. Chances are, it won't be logical or linear and it won't look anything like what you thought it would. Trust what you do know, even if it doesn't seem to make any sense!

EPILOGUE

Anne:

The following exchange between Gary, Dain, and Crystal, a then seventeen-year-old autistic girl, took place in a recent Access Consciousness class.

Crystal (speaking haltingly): I'm Crystal…(breathless) I'm autistic…and growing up…I am blessed to have a family that is super intuitive…I didn't really have to speak…And basically, I didn't for the most part…It's thanks to my grandmother noticing and telling my mom, "You have to teach her how to speak," that I'm even capable of speaking…(long pause)…I have to thank you guys because since Access…my life has really changed…I go out…I have friends …I have a life, I'm starting to really function…

Gary: Yeah!

(Soft laughter and yeah's in the audience.)

Crystal: But there are still times…

Gary: Your mom's crying…(laughter)…She's happy for her kid…

Crystal (breathless):…There are still times when I sort of freeze up …I just can't get to the point of being able to speak in certain situations…or function…

Gary (with great kindness): Can I say something to you?

(Crystal nods.)

Gary: You have extreme abilities, not disabilities, so your inability to talk may have nothing to do with you. It may have to do with other people's inability to hear.

(Crystal audibly catches her breath.)

(Audience applauds.)

Dain: So, I have a question…Is Spanish your first language?

Crystal (without hesitating): I don't have a first language.

(Audience laughs.)

Dain: Au contraire…

Gary: This is your first language. Awareness is your first language.

Class Participant: She also speaks Mandarin, Spanish, and English.

Crystal (smiling softly): And some Danish and some Japanese.

Gary: See what I am talking about—extreme ability? I can barely do Spanish at all and a little bit of English.

Crystal (speaking slowly): My question is…how do I handle those situations?

Gary: By recognizing that when you can't speak, it's because people can't hear. It's not because you can't speak. And you know it. You have a level of awareness that few people on the planet will ever have, and you've got to be willing to acknowledge that. That will give you the freedom to know when to speak and when not to speak.

Crystal: Is there anything I can do then, in situations like that... that people can receive?...I don't want to seem rude...by just not answering people.

Gary: All you have to say is "I'm sorry, I can't answer right now" or "I'll get back to you on that" or "You know what? I have to think about that. Give me a couple of days." By then they will have forgotten and you will be off the hook. You have to learn the lines.

Crystal (laughing): Thank you.

Anne:
Crystal is now studying at a university in Japan.

WHAT DO THE WORDS IN THE CLEARING STATEMENT MEAN?

The Access Consciousness clearing statement is like a magic wand.

Have you ever wanted to be able to just change things by asking them to change? That's what the clearing statement does.

~ Gary Douglas

Right and Wrong, Good and Bad, POD and POC, All 9, Shorts, Boys, and Beyonds

Right and Wrong, Good and Bad is shorthand for: What's right, good, perfect, and correct about this? What's wrong, mean, vicious, terrible, bad, and awful about this? The short version of these questions is: What's right and wrong, good and bad? It is the things that we consider right, good, perfect, and/or correct that stick us the most because we do not wish to let go of them since we decided that we have them right.

POD stands for the **p**oint of **d**estruction, all the ways you have been destroying yourself in order to keep whatever you're clearing in existence. **POC** stands for the **p**oint of **c**reation of the thoughts, feelings, and emotions immediately preceding your decision to lock the energy in place.

Sometimes people say "POD and POC it," which is simply short-hand for the longer statement. When you "POD and POC" something, it is like pulling the bottom card out of a house of cards. The whole thing falls down.

All 9 stands for the nine different ways you have created this item as a limitation in your life. They are the layers of thoughts, feelings, emotions, and points of view that create the limitation as solid and real.

Shorts is the short version of a much longer series of questions that include: What's meaningful about this? What's meaningless about this? What's the punishment for this? What's the reward for this?

Boys stands for energetic structures called nucleated spheres. Basically these have to do with those areas of our life where we've tried to handle something continuously with no effect. There are at least thirteen different kinds of these spheres, which are collectively called "the boys." A nucleated sphere looks like the bubbles created when you blow in one of those kids' bubble pipes that has multiple chambers. It creates a huge mass of bubbles, and when you pop one bubble, the other bubbles fill in the space.

Have you ever tried to peel the layers of an onion when you were trying to get to the core of an issue, but you could never get there? That's because it wasn't an onion; it was a nucleated sphere.

Beyonds are feelings or sensations you get that stop your heart, stop your breath, or stop your willingness to look at possibilities. Beyonds are what occur when you are in shock. We have lots of areas in our life where we freeze up. Anytime you freeze up, that's a beyond holding you captive. That's the difficulty with a beyond: it stops you from being present. The beyonds include everything that is beyond belief, reality, imagination, conception, perception, rationalization, forgiveness, as well as all the other beyonds. They are usually feelings and sensations, rarely emotions, and never thoughts.

WHAT IS ACCESS CONSCIOUSNESS®?

What if you were willing to nurture and care for you?
What if you would open the doors to being everything you have de-
cided it is not possible to be? What would it take for you to realize
how crucial you are to the possibilities of the world?

~ Gary Douglas

Access Consciousness® is a simple set of tools, techniques, and phi-
losophies that allow you to create dynamic change in every area of
your life. Access provides step-by-step building blocks to become
totally aware and to begin functioning as the conscious being you
truly are. These tools can be used to change whatever isn't working in your life, so that you can have a different life and a different
reality.

You can access these tools via a variety of classes, books, telecalls, and
other products, or with an Access Consciousness® Certified Facilitator or an Access Consciousness® Bars Facilitator.

The goal of Access is to create a world of consciousness and oneness.
Consciousness includes everything and judges nothing. Consciousness is the ability to be present in your life in every moment without
judgment of yourself or anyone else. It's the ability to receive everything, reject nothing, and create everything you desire in life, greater
than you currently have and more than you can ever imagine.

For more information about Access Consciousness, or to locate an Access Consciousness Facilitator, please visit:

www.accessconsciousness.com

To find out more about Gary Douglas, Dr. Dain Heer, and Anne Maxwell, please visit:

www.garymdouglas.com

www.drdainheer.com

www.childfamilyplaytherapy.com

About the Authors

Anne Maxwell, LCSW, RPT-S, is a child and play and family therapist, and an Access Consciousness® facilitator. Known as the "Play Lady" by many of the children with whom she works, and as the "Kid Whisperer" by some of her colleagues, she has over 20 years of experience working with children of all ages and backgrounds, who have been given all kinds of diagnoses, as well as with adults and families. Anne now travels the world facilitating classes and has developed a unique approach for change for children and families. She teaches children and parents to tap into and recognize their own abilities and knowing, and to acknowledge that different is simply different; not right, not wrong. And, the results have been magical, phenomenal, amazing! Healing and change are so much easier, more effective, more fun and faster!

Gary Douglas is a best-selling author, international speaker and a sought-after facilitator who inspires people to see different possibilities and to "know what they know." He empowers people to know that they are the source for creating the change they desire and for creating a life that goes beyond the limitations of popular beliefs and conditioning.

Gary pioneered a set of transformational life changing tools and processes known as Access Consciousness® 25 years ago. His work has spread to 50 countries, with 2,000 trained facilitators worldwide. Simple but effective, these tools facilitate people of all ages and backgrounds to help remove limitations holding them back from a full life.

Dr. Dain Heer is an international speaker, author and facilitator of advanced workshops worldwide. He invites and inspires people to more consciousness from total allowance, caring, humor and a phenomenal knowing. He is the co-creator of Access Consciousness®. He has a completely different approach to healing by teaching people to tap into and recognize their own abilities and knowing.

OTHER ACCESS CONSCIOUSNESS®
BOOKS

Being You, Changing the World
By Dr. Dain Heer

Have you always known that something COMPLETELY DIFFERENT is possible? What if you had a handbook for infinite possibilities and dynamic change to guide you? With tools and processes that actually worked and invited you to a completely different way of being? For you? And the world?

The Ten Keys to Total Freedom
By Gary M. Douglas & Dr. Dain Heer

The Ten Keys to Total Freedom are a way of living that will help you expand your capacity for consciousness so that you can have greater awareness about yourself, your life, this reality and beyond. With greater awareness you can begin creating the life you've always known was possible but haven't yet achieved. If you will actually do and be these things, you will get free in every aspect of your life.

Embodiment:
The Manual You Should Have Been Given
When You Were Born
By Dr. Dain Heer

The information you should have been given at birth, about bodies, about being you and what is truly possible if you choose it…What if your body were an ongoing source of joy and greatness? This book introduces you to the awareness that really is a different choice for you—and your sweet body.

Right Body for You
By Gary M. Douglas and Donnielle Carter

This is a very different perspective about bodies and your ability to change yours. It might all be easier than you ever knew was possible! *Right Body for You* is a book that will inspire you and show you a different way of creating the body you truly desire.

Pragmatic Psychology:
Practical Tools For Being Crazy Happy
By Susanna Mittermaier

Everyone has at least one "crazy" person in their life, right (even if it's ourselves!)? And there are a lot of labels and diagnoses out there—depression, anxiety, ADD, ADHD, bi-polar, schizophrenia…What if there was a different possibility with mental illness—and what if change and happiness were a totally available reality? Susanna is a clinical psychologist with an amazing capacity to facilitate what this reality often defines as crazy from a totally different point of view—one of possibility and ease.

Divorceless Relationships
By Gary M. Douglas

Most of us spend a lot of time divorcing parts and pieces of ourselves in order to care for someone else. For example, you like to go jogging but instead of jogging, you spend that time with your partner to show him or her that you really care. "I love you so much that I would give up this thing that is valuable to me so I can be with you." This is one of the ways you divorce you to create an intimate relationship. How often does divorcing you really work in the long run?

Beyond the Stigma of Abuse
By Linda Wasil

If you've tried everything and are still "stuck" or searching, please join me for a totally different way of dealing with the issues of abuse. This book will not be like anything you have previously read, heard or bought as true about abuse. What if this is the information you've been asking for?

Leading from the Edge of Possibility: No More Business as Usual
By Chutisa and Steven Bowman

Just imagine what your business and your life would be like if you stopped functioning on autopilot and began to generate your business with strategic awareness and prosperity consciousness. This is truly possible, except you have to be willing to change. Recognizing a different possibility requires a different mindset and almost always demands a kind of awareness that is not part of prior experience. With this book you'll get the awareness you need to lead your business in any environment!

Joy of Business

By Simone Milasas

If you were creating your business from the JOY of it—what would you choose? What would you change? What would you choose if you knew you could not fail? Business is JOY, it's creation, it's generative. It can be the adventure of LIVING.

CPSIA information can be obtained
at www.ICGtesting.com
Printed in the USA
LVHW040315060919
630167LV00014B/136/P

9 781939 261502